The Politics of Medicare

THE POLITICS

OF MEDICARE

Theodore R. Marmor
University of Minnesota

With the Assistance of
Jan S. Marmor

ALDINE PUBLISHING COMPANY

Chicago

ABOUT THE AUTHOR

THEODORE R. MARMOR received his Ph.D. from Harvard University in 1965 and has taught there and at the University of Wisconsin. He is currently Associate Professor, School of Public Affairs, University of Minnesota. He has been on the staff of the President's Commission on Income Maintenance, involved in policy planning at the Department of Health, Education and Welfare, and closely associated with the research program of the Poverty Institute at the University of Wisconsin. The editor of *Poverty Policy: An Analytical Compendium of Cash Transfer Proposals* (1970), he has published several articles on health and welfare politics.

First published 1970 by
Routledge & Kegan Paul Ltd.
London

Revised American edition
published 1973 by
Aldine Publishing Company
529 South Wabash Avenue
Chicago, Illinois 60605

ISBN   0-202-24036-3   Cloth
       0-202-24037-1   Paper
Library of Congress Catalog Number   76-169517

Printed in the United States of America

Preface

I want to explain the nature of this book and, especially, to alert the reader as to what he may expect in the concluding part, chapter 6. The first five chapters constitute a case study of Medicare politics. This study is not intended to provide a full history of the origins, evolution, enactment, and consequences of Medicare. Those interested in a fuller account of this long, complicated episode in policymaking should consult the studies by Harris, Somers and Somers, and Feingold listed in the bibliographical citations. But neither is this book merely an isolated case study of one important social policy in the United States. Rather, it is both a detailed case study and an attempt to contribute more broadly to cumulative knowledge of U.S. politics and public policy. While these broader concerns are expressed throughout, they are most explicitly raised in the final chapter.

Case studies inevitably mix the peculiar and the typical, the general and the specific, the thematic and the descriptive. By focusing on one decision, one set of government actions, one policy issue, the case analyst cannot "prove" generalizations, but he can comment upon generalizations about politics in at least three useful ways.

First, case studies may be evaluated as instances of particular analytic methods. The notion that such methods lead to selective (and, by implication, biased) analysis can be explicitly evaluated in particular monographs. By reviewing the implicit framework of the study, one can show the respects in which the questions posed, the answers given, and the implications drawn would have differed in other analytic schemes. Such conceptual discussion is important for cumulative work in any discipline; it is the precondition to sustained generalizations from individual studies. Only when units of analysis are the same, central concepts analogous, and inference patterns similar can social scientists "sum up" the descriptions, explanations, and predictions of a number of case studies. Hence, the first respect in which a case study has general relevance (for cumulative effort) is in the explicit discussion of its conceptual framework and the difference such a framework makes in the particular study.

Second, case studies can illustrate some of the problems and prospects of procedural generalizations about political behavior. We have no lack of assertions about how the American political system operates, how public opinion is formed, how concerns become political issues, how legislatures and legislators, executive agencies and executive officials operate in their environments. What we need in many instances is the detailed explication of the connection between such summary generalizations and the innumerable studies of individual instances of political action. A monograph on Medicare —one of the most important post-World War II social policy issues— can be used to illustrate explicitly what seem to be promising generalizations.

Third, case studies can offer important instances of who gets what in the U.S. political system. They can, in short, be used to illustrate generalizations about the substantive content (the benefits and burdens) of U.S. domestic policy. It should perhaps be stressed that Medicare's distribution of benefits and burdens *need* not be typical of domestic, social welfare, or even health policies in the United States. But one can review the Medicare outcome from this substantive-policy standpoint and thus begin to extend the significance of this particular occurrence in American public policy.

All of this can be done without falsely claiming a case study is more than a detailed analysis of how a government behaves in a particular instance. Cumulation of knowledge about U.S. politics will not proceed unless analysts explicitly discuss the conceptual, procedural, and substantive implications of the cases they study.

This book, though not a full history, ranges over the history of Medicare disputes. Three central questions guide its organization and selection of detail. First, why did Medicare arise as a political issue at the time and in the form it did (chap. 1)? The problem is to account for the timing and character of the public policy initiatives we have come to term *Medicare*. The second problem is to describe and account for the pattern of responses to Medicare initiatives over time. The three types of responses include: the nature of the public debate over governmental health insurance for the aged; the kind of group conflict that characterized Medicare; and the sequence of bureaucratic proposals and congressional reactions in the 1952–64 period (chap. 2 and 3). Thirdly, I am interested in explaining the outcome of this intense social policy struggle. The output of the Congress—the Medicare statute of 1965—is the subject of chapter 4. In addition, I set out some of the lessons and issues surrounding the enactment of Medicare. The Epilogue, chapter 5, concludes the narrative by discussing some of the operational problems which arose the first year, and subsequent issues—most prominently the cost increases—bring the book up to the present debate over national health insurance. The last chapter, "Medicare and the Analysis of Social Policy," departs from the sequential organization and reviews the conceptual, procedural, and substantive significance of the Medicare case. Those primarily interested in the policymaking process might benefit by beginning with the last chapter and then referring back to the preceding text.

This American edition carries over the form of documentation used in the English edition (Routledge & Kegan Paul, London, 1970.). Citations in the text, indicated by author's name and year of publication, are fully documented in the Bibliographical Citations section. Following the Citations there is a more general discussion of sources for the study and suggestions for further reading. The Glossary provides further explanation of unfamiliar terms used to describe the legislative process and the medical care and health insurance industries and, under "Abbreviations," a list of institutional names used.

Three institutions have provided support for initial research and forums for criticism of earlier drafts: The Harvard University program in the Economics and Administration of Medical Care; Harvard's John Fitzgerald Kennedy School of Government; and the University of Wisconsin's Institute for Research on Poverty. I want to express my gratitude for such support without in any way holding these institutions responsible for my conclusions.

Full acknowledgment to those who provided valuable and appreciated assistance can be found in the discussion of sources. Jan Marmor was as much co-author of this book as chief research assistant. Her editing has guided the final form of the text and, in many places, her writing has supplied the final version. I want to thank especially the former Secretary of Health, Education, and Welfare, Wilbur Cohen. This study could not have been written without the extraordinary access to primary materials I enjoyed as his special assistant in the summer of 1966. Few young scholars are permitted to investigate the files of political leaders still in the midst of public life. Even fewer are given the freedom I was given to publish the conclusions they draw from such encounters. No one who reads this book will find a slavish devotion to any of my sources, but I feel particularly appreciative to former Secretary Cohen for extending to me the kind of educational opportunity his own teacher—Edwin Witte, the late secretary to President Roosevelt's Committee on Economic Security—extended to him in the heyday of the New Deal.

Allan Sindler, the editor of a volume on *American Political Insti-*

tutions and Public Policy in which a shorter version of this study first appeared, helped more than he realized in making this study more readable. Carol Mermey and Nordis Nesset deserve special mention for so efficiently helping put together the final version of this book for both its English and U.S. editions.

Contents

The Politics of Medicare

Introduction

On July 30, 1965, President Johnson flew to Independence, Missouri to sign the Medicare bill in the presence of former President Harry S. Truman. The new statute—technically Title 18 of the Social Security Amendments of 1965—included two related insurance programs to finance substantial portions of the hospital and physician expenses incurred by Americans over the age of 65. The bill-signing ceremony in Missouri was attended by scores of government officials, health leaders, and private citizens, many of whom had participated in the long, bitter fight for social security health insurance during the administrations of Presidents Roosevelt, Truman, Eisenhower, Kennedy, and Johnson. That afternoon, Johnson reviewed the two decades which had culminated in the Medicare legislation, and observed that the surprising thing was not "the passage of this bill . . . but that it took so many years to pass it."

President Johnson's remark underscored the obvious fact that good health, like peace and prosperity, is a laudable goal, widely shared by Americans. Yet the President was too astute a practitioner of politics to be really surprised by the delay in devising an acceptable federal health insurance program. Public attempts to improve American health standards have typically precipitated bitter

1

debate, even as the issue has shifted from the professional and legal status of physicians to the availability of hospital care, from quackery among doctors and druggists to the provision of public health programs. The beginning of the American Medical Association itself (1847) was part of the broader effort to define the legitimate medical practitioner and to raise the educational standards expected of him. Later in the nineteenth century, licensing of physicians by the states and the regulation of drugs became political issues as the AMA conducted campaigns against medical charlatans and pharmaceutical quackery. Hospital care, once almost exclusively supported by private institutions, became politically controversial once general hospitals grew with the support of local tax funds. Sanitation measures, disease control through mass inoculation, state regulation of hospitals—all commanded increasing public attention as Americans left the countryside to congregate in large urban centers after the Civil War.

It was not until the twentieth century, however, that medical care problems, always of concern to local government, generated interest in national politics. That interest, particularly in the period after World War II, focused on three features of the American system of medical care: medical research, hospital construction, and federal health insurance programs. Since 1945, the federal government massively increased its support of medical research (primarily through the National Institutes of Health, the research arm of the Public Health Service), and under the Hill-Burton Act of 1946, subsidized a significant portion (25–30 percent) of the nation's post-war hospital construction (Somers & Somers, 1961, 50). By 1964, federal, state and local governments together expended almost $7 billion of the $35.4 billion Americans spent in that year for health services. "In few fields," concluded the *Congressional Quarterly* (1, 1965, 1113), "were there more new federal programs established in the postwar era, or more significant changes made, than in health."

Americans were no less concerned about expanding the federal government's role in providing health insurance, but in this controversial area post-war government action did not parallel the rapid expansion of support for research and hospital facilities. The inaction persisted despite public sentiment to the contrary. Opinion surveys from 1943 to 1965 indicated a relatively stable two-thirds majority of Americans favoring some government assistance in the financing of personal health services (Peters, 1946; Cantril, 1952; Hamilton). As proposals became more specific, the public usually showed a less favorable response to any particular method. Yet by 1965, the Gallup pollsters reported, "Sixty-three percent approve of the compulsory medical insurance program soon to be considered by the 89th Congress" (Gallup, 1965).

The legislative activity of the United States Congress, however, is never simply a matter of ratifying public opinion polls. For controversial legislation to be enacted, proponents must be sufficiently organized to make their views felt. There must be some agreement on "remedies" to bolster the public acknowledgement of health "problems." Beyond that, the support of executive agencies is normally required in framing and presenting complex legislative proposals. Bills must have sponsors and floor-managers in both houses of the Congress, and they must pass through a maze of obstacles: committee hearings, placement on the agenda by the House Rules Committee, votes in both houses, and, if successfully passed, a conference committee in which differences between House and Senate versions are ironed out. It was not until 1965 that a health insurance bill for the aged emerged from the congressional process to become public law. Understanding how that bill became law illustrates some of the typical patterns by which divisive public issues run the course in American politics from initial demand to statutory enactment.

1

The Origins of the Medicare Strategy

Twentieth-Century Medicine: The Paradoxes of Progress

In 1912, a distinguished Harvard professor called attention to the remarkable advances in medical science, technology, and therapy which Americans could look forward to enjoying. That year, Professor Lawrence Henderson remarked, constituted a "Great Divide" when "for the first time in human history, a random patient with a random disease consulting a doctor chosen at random stands a better than 50/50 chance of benefitting from the encounter" (Harris, 1966, 5). Twentieth-century developments have fully borne out this prediction that the health industry would have much to offer the consumers of its services. One by one, dread diseases—T.B., cholera, diphtheria, pneumonia, smallpox, polio—have been controlled. Surgical and drug therapy have dramatically reduced the impact of diseases and maladies which preventive medicine has not conquered. These changes, along with substantial improvements in the general American standard of living, have not resulted in diminished illness, but they have startlingly altered mortality rates. The new-born child in 1900 had a life expectancy of 47 years; by 1965 the average was 70 years. These improvements are, however, just

5

one side of what Herman and Anne Somers (1961, 4, 7) have called "the paradox of medical progress." Not only has medical progress increased the proportion of old people in the population, but "as we preserve life at all age levels there is more enduring disability for the population as a whole."

The demand for medical care has increased both through improved capacity and heightened expectations among longer-living populations. Changes in the organization of medical care have accompanied the rapid increase in utilization. Since 1930, the average number of patient visits to the doctor has more than doubled, increasing from 2.6 to 5.3 visits per year. The type of doctors Americans visit has changed in the process. Whereas in 1930, two-thirds of American physicians were general practitioners, three decades later two-thirds were specialists (HEW, 1959). The site of the most complicated medical activity has shifted to the hospital.

With these shifts the costs of medical activities have steadily increased. Between 1953 and 1963, expenditures for all health services more than doubled. The price of hospital beds rose 90 percent while physicians' fees increased 37 percent. The mean expenditure of American families for medical care during this decade grew by 70 percent. Figures on mean expenditures fail to show, however, the uneven distribution of illness throughout the society, and its financial implications. "Much of the total use of health services", a 1967 study concluded, "is accounted for by the relatively small proportion of the population with serious illness episodes"; people with illness "requiring hospitalization account for one-half of all private expenditures, but amount to only 8 percent of the population" (Anderson, 1967, 122ff).

The combination of increased medical competence, heightened consumer expectations and utilization, and rising costs have shaped the environment for public policy demands. But these experiences, common to western industrial countries, have not predetermined either the proposals for government action or their fate. Bismarck's Germany initiated health insurance for industrial workers as early as 1883; England in 1911 incorporated health insurance for low-income workers into a social security program providing pensions, unemployment compensation, and sickness benefits. By 1940, no western European country was without a government health insurance program for at least its low-income workers, though there were substantial differences in beneficiaries, benefits, governmental financing, and regulatory mechanisms. The enactment of Medicare in 1965 illustrated America's comparatively late entry into compulsory health insurance, and its restriction to the aged alone was quite unlike the patterns established in other western industrial countries.

Origins of the Government Health Insurance Issue

Demands in America for government involvement in health insurance date back to the first decade of the twentieth century. The impetus in these early efforts came from academics, lawyers, and other professionals, organized in the American Association for Labor Legislation. During the years 1915–18, this group made a concerted effort to shepherd its model medical care insurance bill through several state legislatures, but with no success. The American Medical Association, whose officials had initially co-operated with the AALL, found local medical societies adamantly opposed to the state health insurance bills, and in 1920 the AMA House of Delegates announced

> its opposition to the institution of any plan embodying the system of compulsory contributory insurance against illness, or any other plan of compulsory insurance which provides for medical service to be rendered contributors or their dependents, provided, controlled, or regulated by any state or Federal government (Feingold, 1966, 89).

Even more disappointing to the labor health insurance reformers was the unequivocal opposition to the model bills of Samuel Gompers, the president of the American Federation of Labor, who feared that any form of compulsory social insurance would serve as an excuse for government control of working men. The strength of the opposition prevented America from following England's example of insuring low-income workers against illness. During the 1920s, a variety of groups undertook studies of health care financing in the United States, and attention turned to the feasibility of group medical practice and of pre-payment medical plans. But it was not until the Great Depression in an atmosphere of general concern for economic insecurity that a sustained interest in government health insurance reappeared. The evolution of the 1965 Medicare Act reaches back to this New Deal period. To understand the particular form of the Medicare legislation, and to explain the two decades of controversy and delay at which President Johnson expressed surprise, one must begin the analysis here.

The source of renewed interest in government health insurance was President Roosevelt's advisory Committee on Economic Security, created in 1934 to draft a social security bill providing a minimum income for the aged, the unemployed, the blind, and the widowed and their children. The result was the Social Security bill of 1935 which, in addition to providing for insurance against loss of income, broached the subjert of a government health insurance program. Edwin Witte, a former professor of Economics at the University of Wisconsin who was executive director of the committee, described the extent of the committee's involvement with health insurance and the critical response of the AMA:

When in 1934 the Committee on Economic Security announced that it was studying health insurance, it was at once subjected to misrepresentation and vilification. In the original social security bill there was one line to the effect that the Social Security Board should study the problem and make a report to Congress. That little line was responsible for so many telegrams to the members of Congress that the entire social security program seemed endangered until the Ways and Means Committee unanimously struck it out of the bill (Feingold, 1966, 91).

Roosevelt's fears that the controversial issue of government health insurance would jeopardize the Social Security bill and, later, his chances for re-election, kept him from vigorously sponsoring the proposal. For many of his advisers in the Committee on Economic Security, however, the discussions in Washington in the mid-thirties marked the beginning of an active interest in the subject. The di-vorce of compulsory health insurance from the original Social Security program of 1935 had alerted the critics within the medical world to the possibility of attempts to enlarge the partial government program, to "get a foot-in-the-door for socialized medicine." In response they reversed their former opposition to private health insurance alternatives: in an effort to forestall federal action, the AMA began to endorse Blue Cross and commercial hospital insurance, and, in the case of state Blue Shield plans, actively to support private insurance plans for surgical and medical expenses (Davis, 1941; Burrow, 1963).* In the meantime, passage of the Social Security Act had freed advocates of compulsory health insurance from pressing concerns about providing income protection for the aged, the blind, and dependent women and children. Their attention was now directed to the broad social question of how equitably medical care was distributed in post-Depression America. From 1939 onward, their activities were reflected in the annual introduction of congressional bills proposing compulsory health insurance for the entire population. An orphan of the New Deal, government medical care insurance was to become one of the most prominent aspirations of Harry Truman's "Fair Deal."

Universal Health Insurance Proposals in the Fair Deal

Although the government health insurance issue was originally raised in conjunction with social security income protection, New Deal-Fair Deal champions of medical care proposals did not view it primarily as a measure to further income security but as a remedy

* The Blue Cross Association comprises non-profit hospital insurance organizations affiliated with the American Hospital Association and its state members; Blue Shield plans, sponsored by state medical societies, are non-profit medical insurance organizations whose boards of directors have been composed mostly of physicians.

for the inequitable distribution of medical services. The proponents of Truman's compulsory insurance program took for granted that financial means should not determine the quality and quantity of medical services a citizen received. "Access to the means of attainment and preservation of health," the 1952 report of Truman's Commission on the Health Needs of the Nation flatly stated, "is a basic human right." The health insurance problem in this view was the degree to which the use of health services varied with income (and not simply illness). In contrast, for those who considered minimum accessibility of health services a standard of adequacy, the provision of charity medicine in doctors' offices and general hospitals represented a solution, and the problem was to fill in where present charity care was unavailable.

The Truman solution to the problem of unequal accessibility to health services was to remove the financial barriers to care through government action. A radical redistribution of income was, in theory, an alternative solution, but not one which the Truman Administration felt moved to advocate. Rather, as he made clear in his State of the Union message in 1948, Truman's goal was "to enact a comprehensive insurance system which would remove the money barrier between illness and therapy, . . . [and thus] protect all our people equally . . . against ill health." Bills embracing such goals had been introduced as early as 1935, but the first to receive widespread public attention was S. 1620, introduced by Senator Robert Wagner (D., N.Y.) in 1939. A decade later, during Truman's term of office, it was S. 1679 which Senator Wagner, Senator Murray (D., Mont.) and Representative Dingell (D., Mich.) presented for congressional consideration. By 1949, the introduction of a Murray-Wagner-Dingell bill had become an annual event which was invariably followed by congressional refusal to hold hearings on the bill.

Through the decade, public opinion polls continued to report favorable reactions to federal involvement in health insurance. However, although from 1939 to 1946 the Democrats controlled both houses of Congress, the partisan Democratic majority did not make up a programmatic voting majority. On the issue of federal health insurance, there were simply too few legislative supporters to bring repeatedly introduced bills through the stages of committee hearings, committee approval, and congressional passage. By 1945, officials within the Social Security Board* had secured presidential endorsement of the Murray-Wagner-Dingell proposal, but the advantage of Truman's support was offset by the congressional elections the following year, which returned Republican majorities in both the House and the Senate. This Congress, it has been observed, "was generally at loggerheads with Truman in domestic affairs," and in the campaign of 1948, the President used its inaction, on health insurance and other domestic issues, to berate the "do-nothing Republican 80th Congress." The election of 1948, returning the presidency to Truman and control of the Congress to the Democrats, left Truman and his advisers with high hopes for enactment of the domestic proposals that had highlighted his "Fair Deal" campaign against Dewey (CQ2, 1965, 4, 7).

Early in 1949, in keeping with his recent campaign pledges, the President requested congressional action on medical care insurance. The specifications of the proposal repeated those of previous Murray-Wagner-Dingell Bills:

—the insurance benefits would cover all medical, dental, hospital and nursing care expenses.

—beneficiaries would include all contributors to the plan and their dependents, and for the medical needs of a destitute minority which would not be reached by the contributory plan, provisions were made for Federal grants to the states.

—the financing mechanism would be a compulsory 3 percent payroll tax divided equally between employee and employer.

* The three key officials—Arthur Altmeyer, Wilbur Cohen, and I. S. Falk—worked in the Social Security Board, a division of the Federal Security Agency. The FSA, created in 1939 to oversee the Board, the Public Health Service, and the Office of Education, was in 1953 replaced by the Cabinet-rank Department of Health, Education and Welfare.

—administration would be in the hands of a national health insurance board within the Federal Security Agency.

—to minimize the degree of federal control over doctors and patients, it was specified that doctors and hospitals would be free not to join the plan; patients would be free to choose their own doctors and doctors would reserve the right to reject patients whom they did not want; doctors who agreed to treat patients under the plan would be paid for their services by the national health board, and the question of whether they would be paid on a stated-fee, per capita or salary basis would be left to the majority decision of the participating practitioners in each health service area (Kelley, 1966, 70, 71).

The bill's reception in the 81st Congress was disappointing to the Truman Administration. Although the Democrats had gained 75 seats in the House, a coalition of anti-Truman Southern Democrats and Republicans blocked most of Truman's major domestic proposals. Despite some success in housing and social security legislation, the federal aid to education bill floundered, and the Administration's health insurance plan was not reported out of committee in either house.

In retrospect, the 1949 campaign for universal government health insurance represented the only time such a proposal had the remotest chance of gaining congressional enactment. The Democrats had their House majority reduced from 263–171 to 235–199 in the elections of 1950, and barely maintained control of the Senate by a margin of two. Attempts to leave doctors' participation in the national health insurance plan voluntary had failed to placate the American Medical Association. The organization had been roused to a nationwide propaganda campaign, directed by the California public relations firm, Whitaker and Baxter, and financed by an emergency "war chest" which was raised by "taxing" every AMA member $25 (Kelley, 1966; Mayer, 1949). The doctors had enlisted hundreds of voluntary organizations and pressure groups to oppose compulsory health insurance, and their crusade was conducted on a note of hysteria, holding out horrific visions of a socialized America ruled by an autocratic federal government. Doctors displayed AMA-provided posters, which presented a color reproduction of the famous Fildes painting of the doctor at the bedside of a sick child. "Keep Politics out of this Picture!" was the accompanying caption (Kelley, 1966, 77). Ignoring the stipulations that doctors would remain free to choose their own patients, and patients to choose their own doctors, the AMA campaign pictured an impersonal medical world under the national health plan in which patients and doctors were forced unwillingly upon each other. In 1950, the AMA took the issue of "socialized medicine" to both the primary and general elections, and their propaganda was credited with the defeat of some of the Senate's firmest supporters of health insurance.

The absence of a programmatic majority in the Congress repeatedly frustrated Truman's health insurance demands. He responded with vitriolic criticism of the American Medical Association as the public's worst enemy in the effort to redistribute medical care more equitably. But the fact was that Truman could not command majorities for any of his major domestic proposals—lambasting the AMA was one way of coping with this executive-legislative stalemate.

Although Truman persisted in requesting compulsory health insurance in 1950, 1951, and 1952, his advisers agreed that after 1949 the prospects for such a broad program were bleak. Among those advisers were Federal Security Agency officials, Wilbur J. Cohen and I. S. Falk,* two of the men who had had most to do with the drafting of health insurance proposals since 1935. Recognizing the need to "resurrect health insurance" in a dramatically new and narrower form, Cohen and Falk worked out a plan that

---

* Wilbur J. Cohen, who in 1965 was Under-Secretary of the Department of Health, Education, and Welfare, became HEW Secretary in March, 1968. Cohen was a member of the staff of the original committee that drafted the Social Security Act of 1935. He was, in 1952, an adviser to Oscar Ewing, the Federal Security Agency head, as was I. S. Falk.

would limit health insurance to the beneficiaries of the Old Age and Survivors Insurance program (the national, contributory, earnings-related pension program for the retired aged and their survivors, established by the Social Security Act of 1935). Oscar Ewing, head of the Federal Security Agency, considered this approach "terrific", and it shaped the entire strategy of health insurance advocates in the period after 1951. The persistent failure of Truman's health proposals had made the need for a new strategy evident; presumptions about the American public's acceptance of social security programs made the content of the new strategy appear politically feasible. Thus the stage was set in early 1951 for what has come to be called "Medicare" proposals. Millions of dollars spent on propaganda, the activation of a broad cleavage in American politics, the framing of choice in health insurance between socialism and "the voluntary way", the bitter, personally vindictive battle between Truman's supporters and the AMA-led opposition—these comprised the legacy of the fight over general health insurance and provided the setting for the emergence of Medicare as an issue.

The Politics of Incrementalism: Turning Toward the Aged

Major shifts in the demands brought to the Congress seldom derive from dispassionate analysis of contemporary social conditions. The decision to pare down President Truman's health insurance aims to a more modest hospitalization insurance program for the aged was no exception to this pattern. In 1951 and 1952 extended discussions took place among Truman's social security advisers about how to deal with congressional reluctance to enact his administration's health program. In October of 1951 presidential assistant David Stowe outlined for Truman three ways of responding to the bleak legislative prospects for general health insurance: "softpedal the general health issue; push some peripheral programs in the area but not general insurance; or appoint a study commission to go over the whole problem." Three days later Truman accepted his staff's recommendation to create a study commission and charged them with finding "the right people" (Cornwell, 1965, 70–71). But the effort to "push some peripheral programs" had already begun, with the President's acquiescence. In June, 1951, Oscar Ewing, acting on the suggestions of Cohen and Falk, announced a new plan to insure the 7 million aged social security beneficiaries for 60 days of hospital care a year. "It is difficult for me to see," said Ewing to an assembled corps of reporters, "how anyone with a heart can oppose this [type of program]" (Harris, 1966, 55).

Ewing, Cohen, and Falk assumed the Administration could most easily build an issue majority in the Congress by narrowing previous demands and tailoring them to meet the objections of critical congressmen and pressure groups. The major objections to the Truman health program which the Medicare strategists felt they had to meet included charges that: (1) general medical insurance was a "give-away" program which made no distinction between the deserving and undeserving poor; (2) that it would substantially help too many well-off Americans who did not need financial assistance; (3) that it would swell utilization of existing medical services beyond their capacity, and (4) that it would produce excessive federal control of physicians, constituting a precedent for socialism in America. In connection with the latter objection, there was the widespread fear, grounded in the bitter, hostile propaganda of the AMA, that physicians would refuse to provide services under a national health insurance program.

To meet these objections, the proponents of "peripheral programs" turned from the health problems of the general population to those of the aged. As a group, the aged could be presumed to be both needy and deserving because, through no fault of their own, they had lower earning capacity and higher medical expenses than any other adult age group. Since the proponents wished to avoid imposition of a means test to determine eligibility within the ranks of the aged, they limited the beneficiaries to those persons over 65 (and their spouses) who had contributed to the social security system during their working life. As an additional advance concession to spike the guns of those opponents who could be counted on to assault the program as a "give-away," benefits were limited to 60 days of hospital care. Finally, physician services were excluded from the plan in hopes of softening the hostility of the medical profession. What had begun in the 1930s as a movement to redistribute medical services for the entire population turned into a proposal to help defray some of the hospital costs of social security pensioners.

The Appeal of Focusing on the Aged

The selection of the aged as the problem group is comprehensible in the context of American politics, however distinctive it appears in comparative perspective. Unlike America, no other industrial country in the world has begun its government health insurance program with the aged. The typical pattern has been the initial coverage of low-income workers, with subsequent extensions to dependents and then to higher-income groups. Insuring low-income workers, however, involves use of means tests, and the cardinal assumption of social security advocates in America has been that the stigma of such tests must be avoided. In having to avoid both general insurance and humiliating means tests the Federal Security Agency strategists were left with finding a socioeconomic group whose average member could be presumed to be in need. The aged passed this test easily; everyone intuitively knew the aged were worst off. Cohen was later to say that the subsequent massing of statistical data to prove the aged were sicker, poorer, and less insured than other adult groups was like using a steamroller to crush an ant of opposition.

Everyone also knew that the aged—like children and the disabled—commanded public sympathy. They were one of the few population groupings about whom one could not say the members should take care of their financial-medical problems by earning and saving more money. The American social security system makes unemployment (except for limited part-time work) a condition for the receipt of pensions, and a fixed retirement age is widely accepted as desirable public policy. In addition, the post-war growth in private health insurance was uneven, with lower proportions of the aged covered, and the extent of their insurance protection more limited than that enjoyed by the working population (HEW, 1964). Only the most contorted reasoning could blame the aged for this condition by attributing their insurance status to improvidence. Retirement forces many workers to give up work-related group insurance. The aged could not easily shift to individual policies because they comprised a high-risk group which insurance companies were reluctant to cover except at relatively expensive premium rates. The alternative of private insurance seemed in the 1950s incapable of coping with the stubborn fact that the aged were subject to inadequate private coverage at a time when their medical requirements were greatest and their financial resources were lowest.

Under these circumstances many of the aged fell back upon their children for financial assistance, thus giving the Medicare emphasis upon the aged additional political appeal. The strategists expected support from families burdened by the requirement, moral or legal, to assume the medical debts of their aged relatives. By concentrating on the aged, the Ewing group believed they could gradually amass widespread sympathy for their plan, leading to a broad agreement that the problem they had defined could be solved by nothing less than congressional action on their proposed Medicare solution.

The same strategy of seeking broad public agreement was evident in the benefits and financial arrangements chosen. The 1951 selection of hospitalization benefits reflected the search for a "problem" less disputable than the one to which the Truman plans had been addressed. General health insurance was a means for solving the problem of the unequal distribution of medical care services; its aim was to make health care more equally accessible by removing financial barriers to utilizing those services, an aim broadly similar to that of the British National Health Service. A program of hospital insurance identifies the aged's problem not as the inaccessibility of health services, but the *financial consequences of using those services*. The provision of 60 days of free hospital care only indirectly encourages preventive health measures and cannot allay financial problems of the long-term chronically ill. The hospital benefit was designed, however, not so much to cope with all the health problems of the elderly as to reduce their most onerous financial difficulties. Ewing and his advisers were well aware that this shift in emphasis left gaping inadequacies. But, in the context of the early 1950s, they took for granted that broader conceptions of the aged's health problems were less susceptible to political solution.

The differences between making health services more accessible and coping with the financial consequences of hospital utilization were continually revealed in the next fifteen years. The statistical profiles of the aged—first provided by the Truman health commission of 1952—uniformly supported the popular conception of the aged American as sicker, poorer, and less insured than his compatriots (Feingold, 1966; Anderson, 1968; Greenfield, 1966). Health surveys reported that persons 65 and over were twice as likely as those under 65 to be chronically ill, and were hospitalized twice as long. In 1957–58, the average medical expenses per aged person were $177, more than twice the $86 average reported for persons under 65 (chart 1). As age increases, income decreases, producing an inverse relationship between medical expenses and personal income. In 1960, it was estimated that approximately "25 percent of the low-income persons in the nation are aged" (Cohen, 1960, 5). While slightly more than half the persons over 65 had some type of health insurance in 1962, only 38 percent of the aged no longer working had any insurance at all. Moreover, the less healthy the aged considered themselves, the less likely they were to have insurance; 37 percent of those in "poor health" as opposed to 67 percent who evaluated their health as "good" had health insurance (Greenfield, 1966). Of those insured aged, a survey of hospital patients reported, only 1/14 of their total costs of illness was met through insurance. There could be no question that the aged faced serious problems coping with health expenses, though it was easy to point out that averages conceal the variation in illness and expenditures *among* the aged.

For those who saw Medicare as prevention against financial catas-

CHART 1

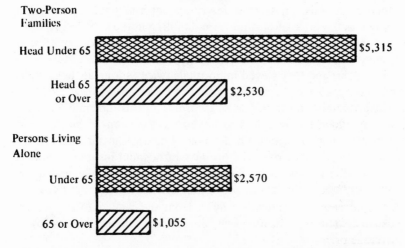

Two-Person
Families

Head Under 65 — $5,315

Head 65
or Over — $2,530

Persons Living
Alone

Under 65 — $2,570

65 or Over — $1,055

Source: U.S. Department of Health, Education, and Welfare, Public Health
Service, *Chart Book of Basic Health Economics Data.* Public Health
Service Publication No. 947-3, Health Economics Series No. 3. Washington, D.C.: U.S. Government Printing Office, 1964, p. 22.

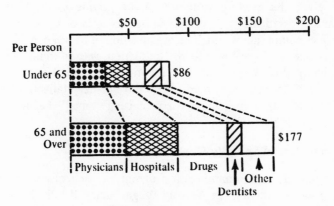

$50 $100 $150 $200

Per Person

Under 65 — $86

65 and
Over — $177

Physicians | Hospitals | Drugs   Other
Dentists

Source: *Chart Book of Basic Health Economics Data,* op. cit., p. 23.

trophe, the vital question was which bills were the largest for any spell of serious illness. The ready answer was hospital care. Not only was the price of hospital care doubling in the decade 1951–61, but the aged found themselves in hospital beds far more often than younger Americans. One in six aged persons entered a hospital in a given year, and they stayed in hospitals twice as long as those under 65, facing an average daily charge per patient bed in 1961 of $35. Hospitalization insurance was, according to this information, a necessity which the aged had to have to avoid financial catastrophe. But what the advocates did not point out was that financial catastrophe could easily overtake 60 days of hospital insurance. Such a catastrophe is defined by the gap between medical bills and available resources. Medicare's protection against the high unit costs of hospital care drew attention away from the financial costs of unusually extensive utilization of health services, whether high or low in average prices.

The concentration on the burdens of the aged was a ploy for sympathy. The disavowal of aims to change fundamentally the American medical system was a sop to AMA fears, and the exclusion of physician services benefits was a response to past AMA hysteria. The focus on the financial burdens of receiving hospital care took as given the existing structure of the private medical care world, and stressed the issue of spreading the costs of using available services within that world. The organization of health care, with its inefficiencies and resistance to cost-reduction, was a fundamental but politically sensitive problem which consensus-minded reformers wanted to avoid when they opted for 60 days of hospitalization insurance for the aged in 1951 as a promising "small" beginning.

Focusing on Social Security Contributors

The financing of the Truman health program had deliberately been left vague by its backers; the Murray-Wagner-Dingell bill of 1949 mentioned a 3 percent payroll tax, equally divided between worker and employer, and administered by a new division within the Federal Security Agency. In the 1951 promotion of a Medicare program, firm emphasis was placed on financing hospital insurance through the already established Old Age and Survivors Insurance system (OASI), enacted as part of the Social Security law in 1935. The use of social security funding was an obvious effort to tap the widespread legitimacy which OASI programs enjoyed among all classes of Americans. But it was a tactic with an equally obvious defect. Proof that the aged were the most needy was based on calculation for *all* persons over 65. Yet social security financing would in 1952 have restricted Medicare benefits to seven million pensioners out of the twelve and one-half million persons over 65. This would have meant not insuring five and one-half million aged whose medical and financial circumstances had been used to establish the "need" for a Medicare program in the first place. Nonetheless, social security financing offered so many other advantages that its advocates were prepared to live with this gap between the problem posed and the remedy offered.

The notion that social security recipients pay for their benefits is one traditional American response to the charge that government assistance programs are "give-aways" which undermine the willingness of individuals to save and take care of their own problems. The Ewing group thought they had to squash that charge if they were both to gain mass public support and to shield the aged from the indignity of a means test. The contributory requirement of social security—the limitation of benefits to those having paid social security taxes—gives the system a resemblance to private insurance. Thus social security members would appear to have paid for hospital insurance. In fact, social security beneficiaries are entitled to pensions exceeding those which, in a strict actuarial sense, they have "earned" through contributions. But this is a point generally lost in the avalanche of words about how contributions, as a Commissioner of Social Security, Robert Ball, once remarked, "give American workers the *feeling* they have earned their benefits" (Ball, 1964, 232). The notion that contributions confer rights analogous to those which premiums entail within private insurance was one which deeply permeated the advocacy of Medicare.

The public legitimacy surrounding the social security program made it an ideal mechanism for avoiding the stigma attached to most public welfare programs. The distinction between public assistance for the poor and social security rights for contributors is, in fact, less clear in law than might be expected. Rights are prescriptions specified in law, and welfare legislation—for any class of persons—confers rights in this sense. But those who insist on the distinction between public assistance and social security focus less on the legal basis of rights than on the different ways in which these programs are viewed and administered. Social security manuals insist on treating beneficiaries as "claimants," and stress that the government 'owes' claimants their benefits. The stereotype of welfare is comprised of legacies from charity and the notorious Poor Laws, a combination of unappealing associations connected with intrusive investigation of need, invasion of privcy, and loss of citizenship rights. The unfavorable stereotype of welfare programs thus supports the contention that social security funds are the proper financing instrument for providing benefits while safeguarding self-respect.

Ewing and his aides were concerned about securing the support of governmental élites as well as organized interest groups and the electorate. They proposed social security financing partly because of the political advantages it offered a president sympathetic to health insurance, but concerned about levels of administrative spending. Social security programs were financed out of separate trust funds that were not categorized as executive expenditures; the billions of dollars spent by the Social Security Administration were until 1967 not included in the annual budget the president presented to Congress, a political advantage not likely to be lost on Democratic presidents worried about the perennial charge of reckless federal spending.

These structural features of the politics of social welfare in America largely account for the type of 'incremental' health insurance strategy adopted at the end of the Truman Administration. They help to explain why the post-war Truman plans of comprehensive government health insurance gave way to a proposal to help defray some of the hospital costs of Americans over 65 who participated in the social security system. Massive public concurrence on the problems of the aged and the propriety of social security was an essential step in the strategy of the incrementalists. Hospital insurance for the aged would have to pass fiscal committees in the Congress where the combined forces of Southern Democrats and conservative Republicans were dominant. The difficulty of extracting social legislation from powerful, independent committees was a lesson which anyone involved in the Truman health insurance efforts could not forget. The strategy of the incrementalists after 1952 was consensus-mongering: the identification of less disputed problems and the advocacy of modest solutions which ideological conservatives would have difficulty in attacking. "In the beginning," recalled Wilbur Cohen, one of the co-authors of the first Medicare bill, "we looked at [the bill in 1952] as a small way of starting something big" (Harris, 1966, 55). The incrementalists, however small their initial demands, were not able to avoid a full, public battle over their proposals once the Congress, in 1958, was moved to hold hearings before the Ways and Means Committee on hospital insurance for the aged.

Pressure Groups and Medicare: The Lobbying of Millions

Serious congressional interest in special health insurance programs for the aged developed in 1958, six years after the initial Medicare proposal. From 1958 to 1965, the congressional finance committees held annual hearings which became a battleground for hundreds of pressure groups. The same intemperate debate of the Truman years (and often the same debaters) reappeared. The acrimonious discussion of the problems, prospects, and desires of the aged illustrated a lesson of the Truman period: the federal government's role in the financing of personal health services is one of the small class of public issues which can be counted on to activate deep, emotional, and bitter cleavages between what political commentators call "liberal" and "conservative" pressure groups. In the press, commentators felt compelled to write blow-by-blow descriptions of pressure group harangues and congressional responses. Within the Congress, clusters of Republicans and conservative Southern Democrats allied to oppose "government medicine" and to declare war against this "entering wedge of the Socialized State." The president of the AMA captured the mood of Medicare's critics in testifying before the Ways and Means Committee in 1963; hospital insurance for the aged, he said, was not "only unnecessary, but also dangerous to the basic principles underlying our American system of medical care" (AMA, 1963, 17).

For all the important differences in scope and content between the Truman general health program and the Medicare proposals, the line-up of proponents and opponents was strikingly similar. Among the supporters organized labor was the most powerful single source of pressure. Organizations of the aged were the result more than cause of these heightened Medicare demands. The National Council of Senior Citizens, formed in 1961 with AFL-CIO financial support, claimed by 1962 a membership of 600,000 (Rose, 1967). The AMA sparked the opposition and framed its objections in such a way that disparate groups only tenuously involved with medical care or the aged could rally around their leadership. A small sample, representing a fraction of all groups involved in the lobbying, illustrates the continuity between the broad economic and ideological divisions of the Truman fight and that over health insurance for the aged (Congressional Hearings 1, 1961):

For	*Against*
AFL-CIO	American Medical Association
American Nurses Association	American Hospital Association
Council of Jewish Federations & Welfare Funds	Life Insurance Association of America
American Association of Retired Workers	National Association of Manufacturers
National Association of Social Workers	National Association of Blue Shield Plans
National Farmers Union	American Farm Bureau Federation
The Socialist Party	The Chamber of Commerce
American Geriatrics Society	The American Legion

Three features of this pressure group alignment merit mention. First, the adversaries who are "liberal" and "conservative" on that issue are similarly aligned on other controversial social policies like federal aid to education and disability insurance. Second, the extreme ideological polarization promoted by these groups has remained markedly stable despite significant changes in the actual objects in dispute, such as the much narrower scope of health insurance proposals since 1952. Proposals for incremental change in a disputed social policy typically fail to avoid disagreement about "first principles." The polarization of pressure groups on Medicare illustrated the typical structure of conflict over "redistributive"* issues in America; the sides, in tone and composition, resembled the contestants in an economic class conflict and framed issues in what Lowi (1964, 707) calls the terms of "class war." Finally, public dispute continued to be dominated by the AFL-CIO and the AMA, lobbying organizations capable of expending millions in the effort to shape the scope of debate and to influence legislative results. Since the 1940s these two chief adversaries have engaged in what *The New York Times* characterized as a "slugging match," a contest of invective. Aaron Wildavsky's description of the conflict between public and private power advocates in America is just as apt for the contestants over Medicare:

[They] have little use for one another. They distrust each other's motives; they question each other's integrity; they doubt each other's devotion to the national good. Each side expects the other to play dirty, and each can produce substantiating evidence from the long history of their dispute (Wildavsky, 1962, 5-6).

The American Medical Association is an organization with conflicting roles. As a type of professional trade union, it is committed to improving the status of physicians. As a scientific organization, the AMA sponsors research and regulates medical practice to im-

---

* By "redistributive" I mean policies which purport to change the distributions of benefits and burdens among broad socioeconomic groups.

prove the quality of health care available to American consumers. As a pressure group, the AMA has fused these roles, linking, and, to some extent, confusing the issues on which physicians speak as scientific authorities and as selfinterested professionals. Its broad lobbying aim has been to convince the American public that physicians are the sole authority that can properly decide on the organization, financing, and regulation of medical care practice. Its major tactic has been to frame the dispute over issues like Medicare so that proponents of federal action meet the widest possible range of ideological objections. The AMA has rallied groups against Medicare behind the slogans of freedom of choice, individualism, distaste for bureaucracy, and hatred of the welfare state, collectivism, and higher taxes. Under such banners have trooped organizations distantly related to health insurance legislation: professional organizations, business and fraternal groups, farm organizations, and various right-wing protest groups.

The mixture of trade unionism and professional activities in the AMA has undermined the credibility of either role. Physicians enjoy both high status and high income (over $34,000 median income after expenses, according to 1964 data from *Medical Economics*). The image of the tireless and selfless practitioner has enhanced the authority of medical organizations in public discourse. Yet recent trends, accompanying the lobbying activities of the AMA, have weakened the claims of medical doctors to disinterested community leadership. Increased specialization (and with that the gradual disappearance of the general practitioner), rising fees, the greater impersonality of medical practice in the modern hospital setting—all have contributed to public dissatisfaction with physicians. The persistent AMA involvement with public policy issues since World War II has increased the risks that an image of the rich and greedy physician will replace that of the noble general practitioner and thus undermine the widely accepted role of the AMA (and its local affiliates) as controllers of medical practice. In these areas, organizations like the AFL-CIO feel less tension; their straightforward championing of the interest of wage-earners means that opponents have little opportunity to dwell upon the gap between the pronouncements of selflessness and the practice of self-interested maneuvring.

Both the AFL-CIO and the AMA have the membership, resources, and experience to engage in multi-million dollar lobbying. Their members are sufficiently spread geographically to make congressional electioneering relatively easy to organize. In 1965, the AMA had 159,000 dues-paying members, and expended a budget of approximately $23 million. The AFL-CIO's 120 affiliated unions represented in the mid-1960s over thirteen million workers; it managed to spend nearly $1 million in the 1964 elections (CQ 3, 1965, 77–78). Both organizations control legally separate political bodies that disseminate propaganda, try to influence elections, and mobilize members for political action. The AFL-CIO's Committee on Political Education (COPE) and the AMA's Political Action Committee (AMPAC—organized in 1961) both spend far more than they report as "lobbying" expenditures. Lobbying—personal contact between organization officials and members of the government*—keeps substantial full-time staffs busy in Washington, but the largest organizational expenditures are for what is euphemistically called "public education." In 1964, COPE's educational tasks cost almost $1 million (*Wall Street Journal,* 1965). In 1965, the AMA spent just under $1 million, of which $830,000 went for the newspaper, radio, and television campaign against the passage of the Medicare bill (CQ 4, 1965; Howard, 1965).

During the debates of the 1940s and early 1950s, the American Medical Association and its allies in big business and commercial agriculture found it a relatively successful tactic to focus the debate on the evils of collectivism and socialized medicine. The narrowing

---

* This restrictive definition of lobbying accounts for the discrepancy between what pressure groups report as lobbying expenses and what they spend in trying to influence public policy. U.S. law (the Federal Regulation of Lobbying Act, 1946) defines lobbying as personal contact between group representatives and officials and only requires that sums expended for that purpose be reported. Hence, the large expenditures for propaganda in the mass media go officially unrecorded.

of health insurance proposals from universal coverage to the aged, however, set new constraints on the anti-Medicare campaigns. In response to the Medicare bills, the aged themselves began to organize into such pressure groups as the Senior Citizens' Councils and the Golden Ring Clubs. Although these groups suffered a lack of the financial and membership resources which characterized the better organized lobbies, it was far more difficult for the AMA to engage in open warfare with them than it had been for the doctors to do battle with the powerful AFL-CIO. When the critics of governmental Medicare proposals seized on broad ideological objections, they now had also to take into account the possibility of being labelled the enemy of America's senior citizens. One effect attributable to this set of circumstances was the appearance of a conservative willingness to offer alternatives. In the late 1940s, Republicans and their allies in the world of big business and organized medicine offered nothing but the *status quo* in opposition to the health insurance schemes of that period. By the 1950s, a change of tactics was in order: it was one thing to write off socialism, but the risks of writing off the aged would give the wise politician some second thoughts.

2

The Politics of Legislative Impossibility

Medicare Under a Republican President

At no time during the Eisenhower Administrations (1953–60) did the Ewing Medicare bills have a chance of congressional enactment. Hospital insurance for the aged lacked the political sponsorship which make controversial bills legislative possibilities. President Eisenhower had campaigned in 1952 against "socialized medicine," by which he meant both the Truman health plan and the more modest proposals for the aged. The absence of presidential sponsorship was compounded by congressional resistance in the tax committees responsible for social security bills (Ways and Means in the House, the Finance Committee in the Senate) where the members were in the main either uninterested or hostile. Among congressmen generally there was not an intensely committed majority disposed to force those committees to report health insurance legislation. Even when the Democrats regained control of the Congress in 1954, the partisan majority did not comprise a favorable Medicare majority. In fact, the legislative prospects were so slight that no committee hearings were held until 1958. "Compulsory health insurance for the general population," it was clear, "declined as a leg-islative issue in the 1950s" (Legislative Reference Service, 1963, 1).

The enthusiasm of Medicare's promoters for future action persisted despite the obstacles of the Eisenhower years. To hasten that future, a group of men who had played important roles in the Truman health insurance efforts pursued their strategy of gradualism. Annually from 1952 to 1960 modest Medicare bills were introduced in Congress, not with any hopes for enactment, but to keep alive the idea of health insurance under social security. At the same time, these promoters turned their energies towards other social reforms. Wilbur Cohen, for instance, director of research for the Social Security Administration until 1956, actively campaigned for disability insurance covering workers over the age of 50. He did so on the assumption that by slowly expanding the number of impoverishing conditions insured against by social security, the risk of catastrophic health expenses would be left as the obvious major omission within the social insurance program requiring remedial legislation.

Once disability insurance was enacted in 1956, the strategists of gradualism concentrated again on Medicare. The four most active members of this group included Cohen, in 1956 about to take up a professorship of welfare administration at the University of Michigan; I. S. Falk, then a consultant to the United Mine Workers; Nelson Cruikshank, head of the ALF-CIO's Department of Social Security; and Robert Ball, a highly respected career official in the Social Security Administration. Their tactical plan was two-fold: to prompt congressional interest in Medicare by persuading a well-placed congressman to sponsor the bill, and to elicit wide public concern about the health and finances of the aged through an AFL-CIO propaganda campaign.

The advocates were successful in both efforts. Although the three most senior members of the Ways and Means Committee rebuffed the Cohen group's entreaties to sponsor its bill, the fourth-ranking Democrat, Aime Forand, from Rhode Island, responded. In 1958, hearings were held on the Forand Bill. Organized labor, which through most of the early 1950s had concentrated on securing health insurance for its members through collective bargaining (Munts, 1967), whipped up a campaign for Medicare in anticipation of the Forand hearings. The hearings prompted the AMA into action as well; it raised its 1958 lobbying budget five-fold, and spent a quarter of a million dollars criticizing the Forand bill. The propaganda battle of the 1940s resumed, with each side matching the other in press releases, speeches, pamphlets, and harangues. Inadvertently, the activity of the AMA assisted its opponents in directing public attention towards health insurance for the aged. Congressman Forand put the point facetiously when he expressed his indebtedness to the "American Medical Association for publicizing my bill so well" (Harris, 1966, 83).

The reopening of extensive public debate did not mean the Forand bill had favorable congressional prospects. In 1959 the Ways and Means Committee rejected the proposal by a decisive margin, in a 17-8 vote. That defeat left many pro-labor congressmen acutely dissatisfied, but their numbers in the last two years of the Eisenhower Administration were too small to force a reconsideration. Yet the aim of renewing interest in social security health insurance had been served. The pressure groups aligned themselves in the "liberal" and "conservative" camps of the Truman years, and turned to the mass media to transmit their continuing claims and criticisms. Future demands for Medicare legislation would be forthcoming— that much was clear at the time hearings were concluded in 1959 and the Forand bill rejected. The question was how would the Congress deal with those future demands.

The Forand Bill vs. the Welfare Approach

The debate over the Forand bill revealed a pattern of disagreement which would continue to limit the alternatives facing the Congress. Both the problems defined as warranting public action and the type of proffered solution remained relatively stable from the time of Medicare's first introduction in 1952. The information gathered on illness, income, insurance status, and health care utilization almost invariably fell into the simple categories of the aged and the non-aged. When Forand's critics attacked his bill, they, too, shared the common focus of attention on the aged. Their argument from the Truman days that all Americans are not poor enough to warrant compulsory government health insurance turned into the argument that not all the aged are poor. That there were substantial health and financial problems among the aged was no longer disputed by the late 1950s. But the extent of those problems amongst the aged, and the means of remedy remained the controversial subjects provoking polarized positions.

The disagreement over the merits of the Forand bill illustrated the persistent divergent approaches to problems of social welfare in American politics. One, the so-called social insurance approach, seeks partial solutions to commonly recognized problems through a financing mechanism that is regressive in character. That is, equal rates of tax are paid by all contributors up to an earnings ceiling, with the result that lower income persons pay a larger proportion of their income in social security taxes than do higher paid workers. It selects beneficiaries not through tests of destitution, but by tests of presumptive need: the orphaned, the widowed, the disabled and the retired are *presumed* to be in need of assistance. Contribution to the social security system thus entails automatic payments of benefits to all those who fall into recognized circumstances of risk, regardless of income.

The alternative approach is that of private and public charity, based on the assumption that most members of a society protect themselves against unfortunate contingencies through savings and insurance. The remaining needs are those of the improvident, the impoverished, and the unlucky, for which the appropriate remedies are private charity, or failing that, local, state, and, sometimes, federal "charity" programs. Levels of payments under these programs are determined individually, by measuring the gap between the financial resources and the needs of the applicant. And the means of financing the benefits are either, in the case of private charity, the largesse of the successful, or, in the case of government welfare programs, the general revenues of the federal treasury and/or state funds. General revenue funding in principle provides a more progressive tax base than that of social security in that, under general revenue taxing procedures, the higher the income the higher the tax that is levied. The social security approach relies upon federal action; the welfare view is that the resort to federal action is the least desirable alternative.

This ideological division revealed itself in the Forand controversy on a variety of issues, but particularly over the questions of who needed help, what aid the needy required, and which financing and administrative mechanisms were most appropriate to the remedy.

(1) On the question of who needed help, the Forand bill specified all the aged participating in the social security system irrespective of their present income. Statistical profiles of the aged which were mustered in support of social security coverage emphasized:

—the high proportion of low-income persons among the aged (U.S. Census data indicated that in 1958, about three-fifths of persons aged 65 and over had less than $1,000 in money income, while another one-fifth received $1,000–$2,000).

—the greater incidence of illness amongst the aged [one indication was the National Health Survey finding that the aged received approximately twice as much hospitalization as those under 65] (HEW, 1962, 22–32).

—the inadequacy of private insurance coverage in meeting the needs of the elderly [social security administrators claimed that 53.9 percent of the non-institutionalized aged were without any form of hospital insurance in 1959, although it was admitted that coverage amongst this high risk group was increasing. Forand backers, however, stressed the shortcomings of private insurance in meeting the total medical costs of the policyholders] (Congressional Hearings, 1965, 40–44).

The critics frequently contested these and similar statistics on the aged, but their main theme was the numbers of aged who enjoyed good health, secure incomes, and private health insurance policies. Conceding that widespread health and financial problems did exist amongst the elderly, advocates of a welfare approach argued that the Forand bill did not address itself exclusively or effectively to those "who really need help," the very poor among the aged.

(2) The problem to which Forand directed attention was the catastrophic effects of large hospital and surgical bills; hence his benefits were limited to those expenses associated with expensive hospitalization and in-hospital medical care. Welfare approach opponents emphasized the inadequacy of surgical-hospital insurance for those whose means had been exhausted and who required outpatient care and drugs. They stressed the need for comprehensive benefits for those aged who could not deal with health expenses through savings, private insurance, medical charity, or state and local assistance.

(3) On the question of administration and financing, the Forand bill called for a federal program financed by social security taxes, emphasizing the contributory nature of OASDI and the desirability of not forcing the elderly to submit to the humiliation of a means test. Many conservative critics, who conceded that federal funds might be necessary to assist the medically indigent aged, nonetheless argued that expansion of federal power was undesirable. A more palatable alternative, to their way of thinking, was to share the financing of any medical assistance program with the states, reserving to the latter the role of administration and of setting standards according to local needs.

Hence, the irony of the dispute: the Forand backers focusing on all social security beneficiaries among the aged, proposing *limited* hospital-surgical insurance for them, to be paid for by *regressive* social security taxes; the more conservative welfare advocates proposing *broader* benefits for a small class among the aged—the destitute —and arguing that *progressive* federal tax revenues should be used, with the administrative organization in the hands of state and local

CHART 2

	Forand Social Security Approach	*Welfare Approach*
Beneficiaries:	Only the aged who were covered under social security	Anyone over 65 whose resources were insufficient to meet his medical expenses
Benefits:	Hospitalization, nursing home and in-hospital surgical insurance (Medicare bills introduced after 1959 specified hospitals and nursing home insurance only)	Comprehensive benefits for physicians' services, dental care, hospitalization, prescribed drugs, and nursing home care
Source of financing:	Regressive social security taxes	Progressive federal income tax revenues, plus state matching funds
Administration and setting of standards:	Uniform national standards administered by the Social Security Administration	Standards varying by state, administered by state and local officials

officials. What led liberals to support the Forand bill was a skepticism that a means-tested, state-administered assistance program would actually be utilized or implemented. Chart 2 illustrates the major differences in approach.

Kerr-Mills Bill of 1960

The welfare perspective on health and financial problems was reflected in three stages. An initial scepticism about the extent of the crisis among the aged subsequently gave way to hope that the substantial health costs of the aged could be coped with by the private insurance industry. Finally, there was a tactical acceptance of the need for federal action. The Kerr-Mills bill of 1960 reflected the conception of appropriate federal responses which conservative congressional leaders felt compelled to offer as a substitute for Medicare proposals. The beneficiaries would be limited to those in severe financial need, but the benefits were subject to few federal limits. Standards of need and benefits would be left to the various states, and the funding would be grants-in-aid, from general treasury funds, to state administrations that agreed to provide their share of the funds for "medical assistance to the aged." These were the characteristics of the bill which Senator Robert Kerr of Oklahoma and Representative Wilbur Mills of Arkansas offered as a substitute for the Forand bill. In 1960, that alternative was adopted by both tax committees of the Congress and ultimately passed as Public Law 86–778.*

The Kerr-Mills program was broad and generous in theory. The federal government would provide between 50 and 80 percent of the funds states used in medical assistance for the aged, with the higher percentages going to the poorer states. Such arrangements, in the opinion of the Senate Finance Committee, would "enable every state to improve and extend medical services to aged persons." The expectation was that the 2.4 million persons on old-age assistance and the estimated 10 million medically indigent would share in the program. Senator Pat McNamara (D., Mich.) was more prescient. "The blunt truth," he told the Senate in August of 1960, "is that it would be the miracle of the century if all of the states—or even a sizeable number—would be in a position to provide the matching funds to make the program more than just a plan on paper." Three years later, McNamara's predictions were confirmed by a report of his special Senate Committee on Aging.† In 1963, 32 of the 50 states had programs in effect, and the provision of funds was widely disparate among the states. Five large industrial states—California,

---

* Wilbur J. Cohen, a life-long advocate of health insurance under social security, wrote much of what became the Kerr-Mills law. Experts like Cohen were so familiar with the localistic, means-test approach to social problems that Kerr and Mills, who both had had long experience with Cohen, rather naturally called him from the University of Michigan School of Public Health to help draft their bill.

† McNamara's special committee was created in 1961 to "make a full and complete study" of "the problems of older people." It regarded the enactment of Medicare as the aged's most vital concern and was a central clearing house for pro-Medicare infomation in the Congress (Vinyard, 1972).

New York, Massachusetts, Michigan and Pennsylvania—were receiving nearly 90 percent of the Kerr-Mills funds, and yet their aged populations represented only 32 percent of the total population over 65 (Greenfield, 1966).

These predictable outcomes did not preoccupy the promoters of medical assistance to the aged in 1960. Both Mills and Kerr were prepared to cope with the worst problem—the health costs of the very poor among the aged—as a way of avoiding Medicare programs in the future. Both were quick to point out that their program allowed for more generous benefits than alternative social security proposals. In a later interview with a national business magazine, Kerr insised on this contrast:

> The Kerr-Mills program provides greater benefits to those over 65 who need those benefits. The benefits include doctors, surgeons, hospitalization, nurses and nursing care, medicines and drugs, dentists and dental benefits—even false teeth. Each state can provide what is needed by the people within the state. The . . . social security approach for aged care would provide mainly hospital and nursing home payments (*Nation's Business,* 1962).

Few states were in fact to provide such broad benefits; by 1963, only four states were providing the full range of care allowed for in the Kerr Mills bill, and most programs imposed strict limitations on the conditions for care and the extent of care (Greenfield, 1966; Congressional Report, 1963). But the program satisfied both those who genuinely believed in the desirability of state rather than uniform national administration and those who hoped even an unsuccessful Kerr-Mills program would head off the demand for Medicare.

The AMA, though originally opposed to the Kerr-Mills bill, soon came to understand its political virtues. In 1961, President E. Vincent Askey, M.D., urged the states to 'implement [the Kerr-Mills program] for the needy and near-needy' (Askey, 1961, 12). Many of the state medical societies did not join in Askey's enthusiasm, but the cause of the AMA's concern was clear. The election of John F. Kennedy, who had pledged to promote enactment of a compulsory health insurance law for aged social security beneficiaries, had returned Medicare proposals to the front pages of the nation's newspapers. In late 1960, Kennedy recalled Cohen to Washington to head a health task force asked to draft a Medicare bill for introduction in the first session of the 87th Congress. When a policy has presidential sponsorship and favorable reactions in public opinion polls, and the partisan alignments in the Congress are supportive of the president, the chances of legislative adoption improve. The election of 1960 thus marked a pronounced shift for Medicare from the politics of legislative impossibility characteristic of the previous eight years to the politics of possibility.

3

The Politics of Legislative Possibility

Medicare, 1961

Kennedy had labelled his platform "The New Frontier," and included within it a variety of proposals for domestic change which he promised "would get this country moving again." As part of the New Frontier, he prominently included a hospital insurance program for the aged. Shortly after his inauguration as president, Kennedy fullfilled his campaign promise. On February 9, 1961, a presidential message to the Congress called for the extension of social security benefits for 14 million Americans over 65* to cover hospital and nursing home costs, but not, in contrast to the Forand bill, surgical expenses. These benefits were to be financed by a one-quarter of one percent increase in social security taxes.

* The 14 million figure was an estimate for 1963, the first full year in which the Kennedy Medicare program could have operated. The projection of 14 million social security beneficiaries, out of a total aged population of 17¾ million in 1963, left an estimated 3¾ million aged uncovered by the Kennedy proposal. The proportion of the aged ineligible for social insurance benefits had been sharply declining since the original Medicare bill. Between 1950 and 1960 the number of aged receiving social insurance benefits more than quadrupled, from 2.7 million to 11.6 million.

39

The New York Times headlined the proposal and forecast a "stiff fight" over the Forand bill's successor. The narrowing of benefits was but one obvious indication that the President and his advisers were aware of the strong opposition to his bill and that they concurred with the strategy long used by Wilbur Cohen. That strategy, designed to modify congressional intractability, softpedalled the innovative character of the program in an attempt to widen agreement on the legitimacy of government involvement in health insurance. "The program," President Kennedy reiterated, "is not socialized medicine. . . . It is a program of prepayment for health costs with absolute freedom of choice guaranteed. Every person will choose his own doctor and hospital" (*New York Times* 1, 1961).

Senator Clinton Anderson of New Mexico and Representative Cecil King of California—high-ranking Democratic members of the Senate Finance Committee and the House Ways and Means Committee respectively—simultaneously and enthusiastically introduced the President's bill the second week in February. Neither, however, was regarded as the pre-eminent Democrat on his committee, and presidents typically try to have controversial bills introduced by dominant figures like Senator Kerr or House Ways and Means Committee chairman Mills. The lesser prominence of Kennedy's sponsors, coupled with the fact that the Kerr-Mills program was in its first year of operation as an alternative to Medicare, left no one in doubt that Kerr and Mills would prove formidable obstacles to the President's Medicare hopes. The ideological composition of the tax committees provided additional basis for skepticism about likely enactment. That the skepticism was well-founded was illustrated by the way in which Ways and Means dealt with the King-Anderson bill.

The Obstacle Course in Congress: First Try with Ways and Means

Kennedy's Democratic majority in the Congress presaged no clear majority favorable to Medicare, and only a majority vote of the entire House could extract the bill from a hostile Ways and Means

Committee. Legislative liaison officials within the Department of Health, Education, and Welfare counted only 196 House members certain to vote for Medicare in 1961—23 votes short of a simple majority. Only an intensely committed majority would even consider the unusual tactic of discharging a bill from committee. The House decision on Medicare thus would rest with Ways and Means.

The composition, style, and leadership of that committee provided ample grounds for predicting Medicare's defeat at the first stage of the formal legislative process. The 17–8 defeat of the For-and bill in 1960 indicated the combined strength of the Southern Democrats and conservative Republican bloc on the committee. Kennedy's Medicare strategists would have to confront this coalition: in 1961, 16 Ways and Means committeemen were known to oppose the bill, including Chairman Wilbur Mills (D., Ark.), whose influence within the committee was formidable. Under those circumstances, the Gallup poll findings that "two out of three persons interviewed would be in favor of increasing the social security tax to pay for oldage medical insurance" (*New York Herald Tribune,* 1961) provided little comfort to President Kennedy. Four votes—either Southern Democrats or Northern Republicans—would have to change for the President to have a Medicare majority within the committee, and the prospects were not good.

The sharp limits on the President's ability to secure the necessary votes are evident in the geographical and ideological character of the House Committee on Ways and Means. Of the 25 committeemen, 15 were Democrats, eight of whom were from Southern or border states. Among the Democrats, there was a clear ideological division between six of the Southern members and the others. *The New Republic,* a liberal weekly committed to much expanded social welfare role for the federal government indicated this ideological-geographical convergence in its annual evaluation of congressional voting behavior. On twelve roll-call votes during the first session of the 87th Congress (1961), *The New Republic* found nine of the Democrats in perfect agreement with the magazine's position. The six other Democrats—all from Southern or border states—voted in accord with the magazine's position 60 percent of the time or less. Among the ten Republicans on the committee, seven were in disagreement with the magazine's position 100 percent of the time; the remaining three, 75 percent of the time. The non-partisan *Congressional Quarterly* studies bear out *The New Republic*'s characterization of a substantial partisan cleavage, with a swing group of six Southern and border state Democrats. Although the *Congressional Quarterly* analyses of the 87th and 88th Congress found Ways and Means Democrats and Republicans to be "more liberal" and "less liberal," respectively, than their party colleagues in the House, the Democratic showing was traced to the nine generally urban, pro-labor members on the committee. Thus, despite the high average support among the Democrats for "liberal" measures, the coalition of ten partisan Republicans and the six more conservative Southern Democrats easily comprised a negative majority on bills expanding the social welfare role of the federal government.*

The conservative coalition opposing Medicare in 1961 was not a happenstance, but a predictable result of the committee's process of recruitment. Democrats on Ways and Means enjoy a unique source of influence, since they also comprise their party's Committee on Committees, the group which makes all Democratic committee assignments. By convention, however, when new Democratic members of the Ways and Means Committee are to be chosen, the Com-

---

* *The New Republic* (1962) evaluation of Ways and Means Democrats, 87th Congress, First Session:

100 percent average approval	*60 percent approval or less*
King (California)	Mills (Arkansas)
Karsten (Missouri)	Harrison (Virginia)
Burke (Massachusetts)	Herlong (Florida)
Keough (New York)	Frazier (Tennessee)
O'Brien (Illinois)	Ikard-Thompson (Texas)
Boggs (Louisiana)	Watts (Kentucky)
Machrowicz-Griffiths (Michigan)	
Green (Pennsylvania)	
Ullman (Oregon)	

mittee on Committees defers the choice to regional party caucuses. For example, during the first session of the 87th Congress, two Democratic openings on the committee occurred through resignation: Thaddeus Machrowicz of Michigan and Frank Ikard of Texas. Their successors illustrated the pattern of geographical continuity: Martha Griffiths of Michigan replaced Machrowicz and Clark Thompson of Texas replaced Ikard. The effect of this customary practice has been to freeze the existing geographical distribution favoring Southern representation and thereby to inhibit additions to the urban, prolabor group among the Democrats.

The nine Democratic liberals in 1961 thus operated in a committee whose structure made their social policy commitments a minority view. Most Ways and Means members enjoy an independence which made it unlikely that the President and the Party could effectively pressure them into changing their votes. Widely regarded as one of the most prestigious House committees, Ways and Means attracts senior and influential members. Members stay on this pre-eminent committee a long time, and are more likely than other repre-sentatives to feel insulated from external pressures. Among the 1961 Democrats, for example, Frazier, Mills and Herlong had served continuously since the Truman Administration and many of the Southern Democrats, including chairman Mills, have run unopposed as often as opposed in their districts. In the 1960 congressional elections, when twenty-one fewer Democrats were returned to the House than in 1958, no Democratic incumbent of Ways and Means lost his seat. Not subject to sharply fluctuating membership, Ways and Means is thus a kind of old-timers' club within the House; its members are beyond the range of pressure from House and Executive leaders which younger congressmen, particularly those who need party help with re-election, may face.

As a rule, the committee is far more responsive to the wishes of the House of Representatives than it is to other sources of pressure. When a bill which is before the Ways and Means Committee has a strong majority on the floor waiting to enact it, its members usually feel a responsibility to report it. When, however, a controversial bill

faces a bitter and close floor fight, the House frequently depends on
the committee to "save it from itself." This gives Ways and Means
the option of not reporting the bill at all or if it chooses to report
the measure, of writing partisan compromises into its first.

The success which chairman Mills has had in satisfying the
House of Representatives is reflected in the reception which Ways
and Means bills have had there. The bills reported by Ways and
Means are generally voted on under a "closed rule," that is, no
amendments are permitted, only limited debate, and acceptance or
rejection. This convention gives the committee great discretionary
power in deciding what to write into their reported bills. House
members go along with the convention because many of them have
neither the time nor the expertise to master the complex technical
details involved in tax, trade and social security bills and because
they prefer to avoid the pressure from interest group lobbies which
those bills generally elicit. Maintaining the closed rule convention
for Ways and Means bills does, however, constrain the committee
to deal responsibly with legislative proposals. Thus, despite the
deep partisan cleavages on the committee, Mills has maintained a
reputation for not allowing partisan considerations to interfere un-
duly with its collective judgment on the technical merits of bills it
handles. When partisan conflict is unavoidable, Mills takes pains to
contain it by compromises which seek to prevent massive Republican or Democratic defections from the bill as it is reported from
committee. The pride which Ways and Means members take in the
regular House acceptance of their reported bills further ensures
their cautious handling of controversial measures like Medicare
(Manley, 1965).

The Southern Democrats

The chairman of Ways and Means had a pivotal role in the fate of
the 1961 Medicare legislation. In less than a year after his own bill,
co-sponsored with Senator Kerr, had become public law, Mills
again faced hospital insurance proposals he had helped to defeat in

the previous session and which threatened now to displace the Kerr-Mills program. At the same time, his influence within the Ways and Means Committee was such that, could he be persuaded to support Medicare, it was likely that he could carry the committee with him.

When it came to dealing with Mills over the King-Anderson bill of 1961, Kennedy was in a difficult position. Medicare was only one of several major items on the Administration's agenda. The President had initiated trade and tax bills of high priority to his domestic program, and these also fell within the jurisdiction of Mills' committee. Since Mills had agreed to introduce these bills in the House, and his support was requisite to their enactment, Kennedy and the House party leaders were at a disadvantage in pressing demands on him to back Medicare as well.

Mills' position in 1961 was affected by an election threat back home. The 1960 census returns required that Arkansas lose two of its six congressional seats, and in the process of redistricting it appeared that Mills would have to oppose Dale Alford in the district which included the whole of Little Rock. Alford was one of the two most conservative and anti-Administration of the Arkansas congressmen. A contest with him would have been the most serious Mills had faced in a House career dating back to the New Deal. It seemed reasonable to suppose that Mills would be disinclined to support legislation, such as Medicare, which in the minds of many Little Rock voters would be too closely associated with an excessive role for the federal government in social welfare policy.

In addition to the chairman, five other Southern Democrats on Ways and Means were opposed to the King-Anderson bill. The President needed at least thirteen pro-Medicare votes to have the bill reported to the floor, and took for granted that none of the ten Republicans on the committee would defect from his party's position. Hence, four affirmative votes were required from among those Southern and border state Democrats who had voted against the Forand bill in 1960.

The 1961 Congress strikingly illustrated a key difference be-

tween the legislative politics of America and those of a cabinet-par-
liamentary system like that of England. Party, executive, and legislative leadership in the U. S. is not, as in England, in the same
hands, and the platform on which a president rides into office need
not reflect the aims of many of his fellow partisans whose assistance
is crucial in the committee and floor stage of the legislative process.
Kennedy's prospects for changing the votes of the crucial Ways and
Means Democrats hinged on the House Democratic leadership: the
speaker, the party whip, the floor leader, and the relevant committee chairman, Mills. While speaker Rayburn was ready to support
the President's Medicare proposal, he lacked formal means to en-
force party discipline on recalcitrant Democrats.

Of the six Democratic opponents of Medicare, Burr Harrison of
Virginia was the least likely candidate for persuasion: a conservative Southerner, he was both fixed in his ways and immune from
pressure. At the other extreme was John Watts of Kentucky. He was
reportedly willing to be the thirteenth vote for the King-Anderson
bill if twelve others could first be mustered; he faced enough anti-
Administration sentiment in Kentucky to make conspicuous support
of President Kennedy a personal liability. Among the other possibilities were the chairman, already a publicly announced opponent,
and Herlong, Frazier, and Ikard, all of whom were at least six-term
veterans of the House and had conservative predilections. Yet,
since they were old acquaintances of speaker Rayburn, they might
have been expected to go along with him in the absence of special
district concerns.

Unfortunately for the legislative fate of the Medicare bill, at the
very time when all the resources and skills of the House leadership
were needed, the speaker himself was in failing health. Majority
floor leader McCormack increasingly took on many of the informal
leadership functions that Rayburn in the past exercised so skillfully.
The Massachusetts Democrat, though thoroughly schooled in the
norms and sentiments of House veterans, could not be expected to
have Rayburn's influence, enjoying neither the speaker's office nor

the immense personal popularity Rayburn, a Texan, had with Southern Democrats of the Watts and Ikard type.

The absence of Rayburn's highly personal legislative management, coupled with the past reluctance of the six "swing" Democrats to support health insurance under social security, meant that chairman Mills' position was unlikely to be challenged within his committee. *The New York Times'* Washington correspondent, Russell Baker, judged this correctly only days after the King-Anderson bill was introduced. "The president's medical program," reported Baker, "despised by many of his own party inside the House Ways and Means Committee, was in great trouble" (*New York Times* 2, 1961).

Earlier in the month, the *Times* had emphasized the equally important fact that Ways and Means faced a "heavy schedule of high priority legislation," with the controversial Medicare bill unlikely to be discussed in hearings until late in the session. The certain opposition of Mills and Harrison, and the probable opposition of the four remaining members of the conservative Southern group, held out dim hopes for those late session hearings (*New York Times* 3, 1961). In the meantime, the problem facing the President was not only to secure these Southern votes on medical care legislation, but to have this group follow party leadership on the foreign aid, depressed areas, tax, housing, and trade bills.

When, as with the King-Anderson bill of 1961, it appears that a committee will not report favorably on a presidential proposal, the president and his allies have alternative strategies. The question facing President Kennedy was whether anything could be gained by any of three possible offensive strategies.

Kennedy could concentrate his bargaining resources on medical care, taking the chance of alienating support on other high-priority bills. Since the outlook for Kennedy's trade and tax legislation was otherwise favorable, both the President and his advisers agreed it would be unwise to press the Ways and Means Committee too forcefully. Moreover, the Democratic margin in the House

(263–174) did not assure passage of the King-Anderson bill even if it were somehow to get to a floor vote: sixty or more of those Democrats appeared unwilling to pass Medicare in 1961. Hence a determined bid for House action was rejected by the President.

The second possibility was to try by-passing the House of Representatives with a Medicare rider to another bill. A rider is a bill which is attached as an amendment to another bill that has already passed one house. In April, 1961, an increasing number of reports suggested the Administration was preparing for a move in that direction. Senator Javits (R., N.Y.), expressed "dismay at reports that the administration had decided to put off a request for Congressional action until next year," and argued that "nothing will happen unless the administration gives [Medicare] priority at this session" (*New York Times* 4, 1961). The support of liberal Republican senators, coupled with broader sponsorship of Medicare among some Democratic senators, led Senator Anderson, Medicare's co-sponsor, to deny late in April that legislative efforts for the session had been abandoned. The proposal was to add a Medicare amendment to the House-approved social security bill then before the Senate Finance Committee.

The Senate Democratic leadership, however, saw strong arguments against the rider tactic. Even if the composite bill passed the Senate, it would be reviewed by a House-Senate conference committee, and Mills' bipartisan influence within his committee was sufficient to force a choice between the social security bill stripped of the Medicare amendment or no bill at all. Kennedy and his advisers discarded the rider alternative, for the time being, and press speculation faded out.

A third option for Kennedy, the one he was to choose, involved accepting the defeat of the bill for that year, but using it to attract public attention to his thwarted campaign pledge. Although he had rejected the use of armtwisting tactics within the Congress, Kennedy hoped to put indirect pressure on legislators by going to the public with an educational campaign about the legislation denied him in 1961. Whatever its short-term effects, that strategy ultimately had prospects of beneficial consequence.

The Kennedy Administration vs. the AMA

Even before the King-Anderson bill was introduced in February, representatives of the Kennedy Administration had begun castigating the AMA for trying, as Wilbur Cohen said at a Washington conference on the aged, "to thwart the will of the majority of the people" by "methods of vilification and intimidation" *(New York Times* 5, 1961). Although clearly the most immediate threat to enactment was the bottleneck within the Ways and Means Committee, it was the AMA and its supporters who drew most of the Administration's fire.

The American Medical Association offered, to be sure, a conspicuous target. Eschewing compromise, the AMA employed every propaganda tactic it had learned from the bitter battles of the Truman era. "The surest way to total defeat," cautioned Dr. Ernest Howard, the organization's assistant executive vice-president, "is to say that the AMA should try to sit down and negotiate" *(Newsweek,* 1961, 103). Instead, AMA-sponsored newspaper advertisements and radio and television spots indicting the King-Anderson bill began appearing throughout the nation. Waving the red flag of socialism, these messages held out visions of a "new bureaucratic task force" entering "the privacy of the examination room," depriving American patients of the "freedom to choose their own doctor" and the doctor of the freedom "to treat his patients in an individual way."

The AMA simultaneously launched less publicized efforts to mobilize local communities against the Kennedy-supported bill. Congressional speeches criticizing H.R. 4222 were reproduced and distributed to newspapers and voluntary organizations. An "Operation Hometown" campaign began, enlisting county medical societies in a variety of lobbying tasks. The AMA equipped local medical leaders with a roster of ready-made speeches, reprints, pamphlets, sample news announcements, a "High School Debate Kit," radio tapes and scripts, and a list of guidelines for using the materials most effectively in reaching "every segment of the American public through every possible medium, [and stimulating] every voter to let his Congressman know that medicare is really 'Fedicare'—a costly concoction of bureaucracy, bad medicine, and an unbalanced budget" (AMA, 1961).

As conspicuous as the AMA was in criticism, the Administration's effort to confront the organization indicated the legislative frustration awaiting Medicare. Since King-Anderson supporters could do little to bring direct pressure on the pivotal congressmen in Ways and Means, they hoped their representation of the AMA as an unscrupulous and inordinately powerful interest which was successfully thwarting the public would cause congressional critics of Medicare to suffer guilt by association. In April, Health, Education, and Welfare Secretary Abraham Ribicoff debated Senator Kenneth Keating (R., N.Y.) on television over the King-Anderson bill, and used the opportunity to lash out against the "scare tactics" of "organized medicine's" campaign against compulsory health insurance for the aged (*New York Times* 6, 1961).

The Ways and Means hearings of July and August provided another prominent occasion for continuing the bid for public support. The testimony of representatives from HEW linked the well-known case for the King-Anderson bill to a blistering attack on the pressure groups opposing it. The Administration spokesmen, along with those of the AFL-CIO, diverted their attention from the specifications of the Medicare bill to the methods and interests of their medical, business, and hospital critics. The testimony of Secretary Ribicoff attempted to discredit AMA predictions of creeping socialism and the end of freedom by outlining again the modest character of Medicare. "The bill is designed," he said,

only to take care of the aged. It is not my intention to advocate that we take care of the medical needs and hospital needs of our entire population, and the reason is that insurance is available for younger people. Blue Cross is available and it can be paid for by working population (Congressional Hearings 2, 1961).

Ribicoff stressed the two characteristics which most sharply distinguished English from American debates over government health activities. No hope was expressed of divorcing health care from consideration of finances, but only of taking care of a group with special problems in purchasing private insurance. Even the insurance was only to cover "unusual hospital needs", leaving out drugs, doctors' fees, and a whole range of other medical expenses. This raises the second point: the fact that the terms of the debate—the issues which proponents of the King-Anderson bill had to face—had been set by the opponents in the medical world. This pattern continued throughout the hearings, with the exception of the Socialist Party's representative, who industriously tried to point out how modest and inadequate the proposed bill really was.

The press gave prominent coverage to the summer hearings, but the behavior of the committee members indicated that the bill's fate was a foregone conclusion. The Southern Democrats, whose views were central to the committee outcome, were relatively quiet. Chairman Mills, who ordinarily took a dominant role in executive hearings on major bills, missed two of the nine open sessions, and remained dispassionate during most of those he chaired. Questioning was left primarily to a few of the anti-Medicare Republicans and pro-Medicare Democrats who were amenable to joining the propaganda battle being waged by those giving testimony.

At the end of nine days, on August 4, 1961, the hearings ended undramatically. A week later *The New York Times* reported that no further action on the King-Anderson bill was contemplated for that session. Amidst the national concern over Berlin and the call-up of reserve units, many Americans were unaware of the fate of what had been a campaign issue, or of the fact that Ways and Means had failed even to take a formal vote on the bill. Chairman Mills, unwilling as ever to highlight the partisan cleavages within

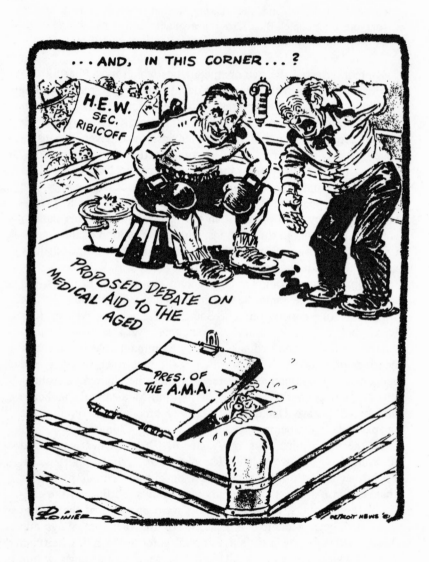

the committee, and sharing with his fellow committeemen, and congressmen generally, a reluctance to clarify their public record with anything so concrete as a yes or no vote when there was little to be gained by it, preferred to let the bill die an anonymous death. If future events should force a reconsideration of the committee's position on Medicare—and Mills was aware of the possibility—a telltale 1961 vote might prove an embarrassment. Nor did the Kennedy Administration, with an interest in future negotiations with Ways and Means, wish to burden Medicare with the legacy of a negative vote. The quietness of Medicare's burial made it easier for the bill's supporters to blame its murder on the AMA while diverting attention from the active complicity of the House committee and the passive complicity of the Kennedy Administration.

Some analysts of American politics have confused Medicare defeats of the 1961 variety with AMA victories. "Measures apparently assured of passage," according to a *Yale Law Journal* study (1954, 995), "have been voted down, buried in committee, or substantially amended, upon the announcement of AMA disapproval." The AMA is thus pictured as a supreme legislative string-puller, the "only organization that could marshal 140 votes in Congress between sundown Friday night and noon Monday morning." Neglected in this stereotyped portrait is the distinction between results the AMA approves (or disapproves) and those they produce. The AMA has few resources for coercing individual congressmen to change their votes, especially senior, autonomous figures on committees like Ways and Means. That a coalition within the committee shared some of the AMA's ideological predispositions should not lead one to assume that the AMA controlled the votes.

This is not to say the efforts of pressure groups opposed to Medicare were unimportant, but rather that they were important in other ways. The AMA and its ideological allies brought the issue to public view in terms likely to place Medicare advocates on the defensive. Their impact was evident in the character of debate over medical care for the aged and especially in the narrowing of Medicare proposals to exclude coverage of physicians' care. But to account for the 1961 legislative outcome, one must turn from the public debate to the internal character of the Committee on Ways and Means. Only by doing so can one explain why the Medicare bill, initiated by the President and acceptable to a majority of Americans polled on the issue, could be undramatically defeated at the committee stage of the legislative process.

Medicare's Near Miss, 1964

Between the defeat of President Kennedy's initial Medicare proposal in 1961 and the national elections of 1964, none of the major congressional obstacles to its enactment were fully removed. The Democrats maintained control of the Congress after the 1962 elections, but the pro-Administration bloc was, as usual, never as large as the number of Democrats. In 1961, HEW's congressional liaison staff estimated the House Medicare breakdown as approximately twenty-three votes short of a 218 majority. The Ways and Means Committee never gave them the chance to check the accuracy of their estimates, and attempts to circumvent the committee with rider strategies proved abortive in 1962 and 1964. Each year hearings were held on Medicare, and by 1964, thirteen volumes of testimony had been compiled, totalling nearly 14,000 pages. But Wilbur Mills and his committee were not ready to report a Medicare bill.

The Administration's pro-Medicare strategy included continued efforts to change votes on the committee. Two methods were employed. First, HEW officials were directed to respond to the objections of the key Southern Democrats in hopes of bringing them around on the King-Anderson bill. When HEW Assistant Secretary Wilbur Cohen was informed of President Kennedy's assassination on November 22, 1963, he was in the midst of preparing changes in the Administration bill which would answer some of Mills' criticisms. Cohen and his staff spent far more time courting critics than they did working with pro-Medicare members of the committee. The Administration, through the influence of House Democratic leadership over members of the regional caucusses, also took steps to enlarge the size of the pro-Medicare group. After 1961, no new member of the committee was elected who had failed to assure the House leadership that he would vote for Medicare or, at the very least, would support its being reported out of the Ways and Means Committee. By 1964, these efforts had brought the total of pro-Medicare Democrats to twelve, one short of a committee majority. Three of the anti-Medicare Southern Democrats of 1961, Frazier, Harrison and Ikard had been replaced by fellow Southerners who were willing to support the King-Anderson bill, Richard Fulton, Pat Jennings and Clark Thompson, the latter the most reluctant. All the other Democratic newcomers between 1961 and 1964 were, like their predecessors, firm Administration supporters.

This weakening of the anti-Medicare coalition revealed both the opportunities and risks which the politics of legislative possibility entail for Democratic reformers. Sensing victory within the Senate and realizing the narrow margin enjoyed by Medicare opponents within Ways and Means, President Johnson and congressional leaders thought again of a rider amendment in the Senate. But Ways and Means opponents were equally aware of the changed probabilities and nearly pulled off a clever legislative coup in the early summer of 1964. The senior Republican, John W. Byrnes of Wisconsin, proposed that the 5 percent increase in social security benefits which the committee had approved in earlier deliberations be increased to 6 percent. This would have raised social security taxes to 10 percent, widely accepted within Congress at that time as the upper social insurance tax limit, and thus leave no fiscal room for Medicare in the future. The pro-Medicare committeemen realized the trap, but only 11 of their number were at the roll call vote. The anti-Medicare group seemed to have a winning margin, 12–11. But the final vote cast was by Bruce Alger, an arch-conservative Republican from Dallas. Unwilling to play the game, Alger voted with the Democratic majority, explaining later that "since he opposed the entire Social Security system, consistency would not permit him to expand it," even to undermine the chances of Medicare (Harris, 1966, 164).

Having observed their House brethren come close to catastrophe, Senate Democrats acted to attach the Medicare rider to the social security bill which the House had already passed in 1964. But Mills had anticipated that move and, fearing that Ways and Means would lose control over the content of any Medicare bill, had taken steps to thwart it. He promised pro-Medicare Democrats on his committee that Medicare would be the "first order of business" in 1965; in return he received their support in rejecting the rider in the conference committee. With the House and Senate Republican conferees already anxious to stop Medicare, Mills had enough votes to accomplish this task. On October 4, the conference announced its deadlock over the entire social security bill, thus postponing both the social security cash benefit increases and Medicare until the following year.

The circumstances of Medicare's defeat in the fall of 1964 illustrated how substantially the possibilities of enactment had increased since the first Kennedy effort in 1961. The Senate was on record favoring the King-Anderson bill and the key bottleneck of 1961, the Ways and Means Committee, was within one vote of a health insurance majority. Wilbur Mills' promises for 1965 evidenced the weakened position of the anti-Medicare coalition. In September and December of 1964, Mills suggested to audiences in Little Rock that a soundly financed Medicare bill would gain his support in the next session of the Congress. Having already stated that medical care insurance would be the first order of business for his committee the following January, Mills expressed his concerns about the discrepancies between popular conceptions of Medicare and the content of the King-Anderson proposals. "The public," Mills warned in his Little Rock speech of December 7, "must be under no illusion regarding the benefits . . . [and must understand that] Medicare does not refer to doctor services' or general outpatient medical care" (Mills, 1964).

Mills' worry was not ill-founded. "Medicare," a term which originally referred to the comprehensive health program run for servicemen's families by the Defense Department, was a misleading slogan for the King-Anderson bill. "Hospicare" would have been a more appropriate epithet. Despite the accretion of support between 1961 and 1964, the King-Anderson bills had changed only slightly. After 1963, Medicare was altered to include non-social security beneficiaries for a limited period, and here and there changes were made in the level of benefits. But the bill over which the conference committee deadlocked in 1964 remained basically a hospital insurance measure. When the deadlock was announced, observers, taking their cue from Mills' promises, assumed the King-Anderson proposal would be close to passage in 1965. In the meantime, the election of November, 1964, changed practically every political consideration; and Mills' ruminations in December about the unrealistic conception Americans held of Medicare was the first sign that anyone read the striking electoral victory of the Democrats to mean anything more than speedy enactment of a bill providing hospitalization and nursing home insurance for the aged. The *Congressional Quarterly* (5, 1965) soberly observed that "some type of medical care program for the aged is expected to be enacted by Congress in 1965."

4

The Politics of Legislative Certainty

The Impact of the Election of 1964

The electoral outcome of 1964 guaranteed the passage of legislation on medical care for the aged. Not one of the obstacles to Medicare was left standing. In the House, the Democrats gained thirty-two new seats, giving them a more than two-to-one ratio for the first time since the heyday of the New Deal. In addition, President Johnson's dramatic victory over Goldwater could be read as a popular mandate for Medicare. The President had campaigned on the promise of social reforms—most prominently Medicare and federal aid to education—and the public seemed to have rejected decisively Goldwater's alternatives of state, local, and private initiative.

Within the Congress, immediate action was taken to prevent the use of delaying tactics previously employed against both federal aid to education and medical care bills. Liberal Democratic members changed the House rules so as to reduce the power of Republican-Southern Democratic coalitions on committees to delay legislative proposals. The twenty-one-day rule was reinstated, making it possible to dislodge bills from the House Rules Committee after a maximum delay of three weeks.

At the same time changes affecting the Ways and Means Committee were made which reduced the likelihood of further efforts to delay Medicare legislation. The traditional ratio of three members of the majority party to two of the minority party was abandoned for a ratio reflecting the strength of the parties in the House as a whole (two-to-one). In 1965, that meant the composition of Ways and Means shifted from fifteen Democrats and ten Republicans to seventeen Democrats and eight Republicans, insuring a pro-Medicare majority. A legislative possibility until the election of 1964, the King-Anderson program had become a statutory certainty. The only question remaining was the precise form the health insurance legislation would take.

The Administration's Proposal: H.R. 1 and S. 1

Administration leaders assumed after the election that the Ways and Means Committee would report a bill similar to the one rejected by the conference in 1964. Hence Anderson and King introduced on January 4, 1965, in the Senate and House respectively, the standard Medicare package: coverage of the aged, limited hospitalization and nursing home insurance benefits, and social security financing. The HEW staff prepared a background guide on the bill which continued to emphasize its modest aims. The guide included assurances that the bill's coverage of hospitalization benefits "left a substantial place for private insurance for nonbudgetable health costs, [particularly for] physicians' services." It described H.R. 1 as "Hospital Insurance for the Aged through Social Security," and no doubt would have encouraged the substitution of "Hospicare" for "Medicare" as its popular name, had this been still possible by 1965 (HEW 1, 1965).

Social security experts within HEW, with a rich history of sponsoring unsuccessful health insurance bills, were doubly cautious now that success seemed so near at hand. Wilbur Cohen, for instance, busied himself, with President Johnson's blessings, convincing the congressional leadership to give Medicare the numerical symbol of highest priority among the President's Great Society proposals: hence Medicare became H.R. 1 and S. 1. Its content, however, remained essentially unchanged. The HEW leaders, like everyone else, could read the newspapers and find criticisms that Medicare's benefits were insufficient, and that the aged mistakenly thought the bill covered physicians' services. The strategists believed, however, that broader benefits—such as coverage of physicians' care—could wait: the reformers' fundamental premise had always been that Medicare was only "a beginning," with increments of change set for the future.

The election of 1964 had a vastly different impact on critics of Medicare than on promoters of the Administration bill, H.R. 1. If the election promoted satisfaction among H.R. 1's backers with their customary position, it provoked significant reactions among its opponents. Both Republican and AMA spokesmen shifted to discussions of what one AMA official, Dr. Ernest Howard, called "more positive programs". These alternatives grew out of the familiar criticisms that the King-Anderson bills had "inadequate" benefits, would be too costly, and made no distinction between the poor and wealthy among the aged. The AMA gave the slogan "Eldercare" to its bill, and had it introduced as H.R. 3737 by Thomas Curtis (R., Mo.) and A. Sydney Herlong (D., Fla.), both Ways and Means members. In comparing its bill and H.R. 1, the AMA earnestly stressed the disappointingly limited benefits of the latter:

> Eldercare, implemented by the states would provide a wide spectrum of benefits, including physicians' care, surgical and drug costs, nursing home charges, diagnostic services, x-ray and laboratory fees and other services. Medicare's benefits would be far more limited, covering about one-quarter (25 percent) of the total yearly health care costs of the average person. . . . Medicare would *not* cover physicians' services or surgical charges. Neither would it cover drugs outside the hospital or nursing home, or x-ray or other laboratory services not connected with hospitalization (AMA, 1965).

Claiming their "program offered more benefits for the elderly at less cost to the taxpayers," the AMA charged, as did some Republicans, that the public had been misled by the connotations of the "Medicare" epithet. Seventy-two percent of those questioned in an AMA-financed survey during the first two months of 1965 agreed that doctors' bills should be insured in a government health plan. Sixty-five percent of the respondents preferred a selective welfare program which would "pay an elderly person's medical bill only if he were in need of financial help" to a universal social security plan which would "pay the medical expenses of everyone over 65 regardless of their income." Armed with these figures, the AMA once again launched a full-scale assault on the King-Anderson bill, hoping to head it off with what amounted to an extension of the Kerr-Mills program.

By February, the issue was once again before the Ways and Means Committee. Pressure groups—medical, labor, hospital and insurance organizations primarily—continued to make public appeals through the mass media and made certain their viewpoints were presented to the committee. Ways and Means had before it three legislative possibilities: the Administration's H.R. 1, the AMA's Eldercare proposal, and a new bill sponsored by the senior Republican committee member, John Byrnes.

The Ways and Means Committee and the House Take Action: January-April

For more than a month Ways and Means worked on H.R. 1, calling witnesses, requesting detailed explanation of particular sections, and trying to estimate its costs and benefits. Executive sessions, closed to the press and one mark of serious legislative intent, began in January. The atmosphere was business-like and deliberate; members assumed the Administration bill would pass, perhaps with minor changes, and there was little disposition to argue the broad philosophical issues that had dominated hearings in the preceding decade. When spokesmen for the AMA invoked their fears of socialized medicine, they irritated committee members intent on working out practical matters, and chairman Mills refused to consult AMA representatives in further sessions of the committee's officially unreported deliberations.

Mills led his committee through practically every session of hearings on the Administration bill, promising to take up the Byrnes bill (H.R. 4351) and the Eldercare bill in turn. By March 1, there had been continued reference to the exclusions and limits of the King-Anderson bill, with the charges of inadequacy coming mostly from the Republicans. On March 2, announcing his concern for finding "some degree of compromise [that] results in the majority of us being together," Mills invited Byrnes to explain his bill to the committee.

The Byrnes bill was ready for discussion because the Republicans on the committee, in the wake of the 1964 election, wanted to prevent the Democrats from taking exclusive credit for a Medicare law. The Republican staff counsel, William Quealy, had explained this point in a confidential memorandum in January, reminding the Republican committeemen that they had to "face political realities." Those realities included the certain passage of health insurance legislation that session and excluded the strategy of substituting an expanded Kerr-Mills program. "Regardless of the intrinsic merits of the Kerr-Mills program," Quealy (1965) wrote, "it has not been accepted as adequate . . . particularly by the aged, [and a] liberalization of it will not meet the political problem facing the Republicans in this Congress." That problem was the identification of Republicans with diehard AMA opposition to Medicare, which some Republican leaders thought contributed heavily to their 1964 electoral catastrophe. Hence Byrnes, who had been working since January on a Republican alternative, was anxious to distinguish his efforts from those of the AMA. At the same time, with the AMA spending nearly $900,000 to advertise its Eldercare plan, the criticism of H.R. 1's "inadequacies" was given wide circulation.

Byrnes emphasized that his bill, which proposed benefits similar to those offered in the Aetna Life Insurance Company's health plan for the federal government's employees, would cover the major risks overlooked by H.R. 1, particularly the costs of doctors' services and drugs. He also stressed the voluntary nature of his proposal; the aged would be free to join or not, and their share of the financing would be "scaled to the amounts of the participants' social security cash benefits," while the government's share would be drawn from general revenues (Cohen and Ball, 1965, 5). The discussion of the Byrnes bill was spirited and extended; the AMA's Eldercare alternative, not promoted vigorously by even its committee sponsors, was scarcely mentioned.

The Byrnes and King-Anderson bills were presented as mutually exclusive alternatives. HEW officials were exhausted from weeks of questioning and redrafting, and viewed the discussion of the Byrnes bill as a time for restful listening. But Mills, instead of posing a choice between the two bills, unexpectedly suggested a combination which involved extracting Byrnes' benefit plan from his financing proposal. On March 2, Mills turned to HEW's Wilbur Cohen and calmly asked whether such a "combination" were possible. Cohen was "stunned," and initially suspicious that the suggestion was a plot to kill the entire Administration proposal. No mention had even been made of such innovations. Cohen had earlier argued for what he called a "three-layer cake" reform by Ways and Means: H.R. 1's hospital program first, private health insurance for physician's coverage, and an expanded Kerr-Mills program "underneath" for the indigent among the aged. Mills' announcement that the committee appeared to have "gotten to the point were it is possible to come up with a medi-elder-Byrnes bill" posed a surprise possibility for a different kind of combination. That night, in a memorandum to the President, Cohen reflected on Mills' "ingenious plan," explaining that a proposal which put "together in one bill features of all three of the major" alternatives before the committee would make Medicare "unassailable politically from any serious Republican attack" (Cohen, 1965). Convinced now that Mills' strategy was not destructive, Cohen was delighted that the

Republican charges of inadequacy had been used by Mills to prompt the expansion of H.R. 1.

Byrnes himself was reluctant to approve the dissection of his proposal, humorously referring to his bill as "better-care." Nonetheless, from March 2 to March 23, when the committee finished its hearings, Ways and Means members concentrated on the combination of what had been mutually exclusive solutions to the health and financial problems of the elderly. Mills presided over this hectic process with confident but gracious assurance, asking questions persistently but encouraging from time to time comments from other members, especially from the senior Republican, Byrnes. The Byrnes benefit formula was slightly reduced; the payment for drugs used outside hospitals and nursing homes, for instance, was rejected on the grounds of unpredictable and potentially high costs. After some consideration of financing the separate physicians' insurance through social security, the committee adopted Byrnes' financing suggestion of individual premium payments by elderly beneficiaries, with the remainder drawn from general revenues. But while Byrnes had proposed that such premiums be scaled to social security benefits, the committee prescribed a uniform $3 per month contribution from each participant. The level of premium was itself a matter of extended discussion: HEW actuaries estimated medical insurance would cost about $5 per month, but Mills cautiously insisted that a $6 monthly payment would make certain that expenditures for medical benefits were balanced by contributions *(Congressional Report* 1, 1965).

HEW was of course vitally interested in the uses to which Mills put the Byrnes plan. As one of the chief HEW participants, Irwin Wolkstein, explained (1968),

Many features of the Byrnes Bill which had been objectionable were changed to be sure to keep administration support although some objections remained—including inadequate protection of beneficiaries against over-charging, absence of quality standards, and carrier responsibility for policy. The issue to the Department was whether the benefit advantages to the aged of SMI [Supplementary Medical Insurance] overweighed the dificiencies, and the answer of the administration was yes.

In its transformation into the "first layer" of the new "legislative cake," H.R. 1 was not radically altered. Levels of particular benefits were changed, reducing, among other things, the length of insured hospital care, and increasing the amount of the hospital deductible and co-insurance payment beneficiaries would have to pay. (Deductibles are the payments patients must make before their insurance takes over, and co-insurance contributions are the proportion of the remaining bill for which patients are responsible.) The continuing debate over these matters illustrated the divergent goals of those involved in reshaping Medicare. High deductibles but no limit on the number of insured hospital days were sought by those anxious to provide protection against chronic and catastrophic illness. Others insisted on co-insurance and deductibles so that patients would be given a stake in avoiding overuse of hospital facilities. But the most contested changes made in H.R. 1 involved the methods of paying hospital-based RAPP specialists (radiologists, anaesthetists, pathologists, and physiatrists) and the level of increase in social security taxes required to pay for the hospitalization plan.

The Johnson Administration recommended that the charges for services like radiology and anaesthesiology be included in hospital bills unless existing hospital-specialist arrangements called for another form of payment. Mills, however, insisted that "no physician service, except those of interns and residents under approved teaching programs, would be paid" under H.R. 1, now Part A of the bill Mills had renumbered H.R. 6675. His provision required changes in the customary billing procedure of most hospitals, and became the subject of bitter disagreement. Such an arrangement, hospital officials quickly reminded the committee, would cause administrative difficulties and upset existing arrangements. But Mills stuck by his suggestion and easily won committee approval. More than any other issue, the method of paying these hospital specialists was to plague efforts in the Senate and conference committee to find a compromise version of the bill Mills steered through the Ways and Means Committee and the House.

Ways and Means also required more cautious financing of the hospital program than the Administration suggested. Social Security taxes—and the wage base on which those taxes would be levied— were increased so as to accommodate even extraordinary increases in costs. The final committee report announced with some pride that their estimates of future hospital benefits reflected a "more conservative basis than recommended by the [1964 Social Security] Advisory Council and, in fact, more conservative than those used by the insurance industry in its estimates of proposals of this type" *(Congressional Report* 2, 1965, 54). (Mills' penchant for "actuarial soundness" was justified by Medicare's costs during the first year of operation; in 1966 both hospital and physician charges more than doubled their past average rate of yearly increase, thus substantially inflating program costs beyond HEW's initial predictions (HEW 1, 1967).)

Throughout March, Mills called on committee members, HEW officials, and interest group representatives to lend their aid in drafting a combination bill. The advice of the Blue Cross and American Hospital Associations was taken frequently on technical questions about hospital benefits. HEW spokesmen were asked to discuss many details with directly interested professional groups and report back their findings. Blood bank organizations, for instance, were consulted on whether Medicare's insurance of blood costs would hamper voluntary blood-giving drives. Their fear that it would, prompted the committee to require that Medicare beneficiaries pay for or replace the first three pints of blood used during hospitalization. Throughout, Mills left no doubt that he was first among equals—he acted as the conciliator, the negotiator, the manager of the bill, always willing to praise others, but guiding the "marking up" of H.R. 6675 through persuasion, entreaty, authoritative expertise, and control of the agenda.

The Medicare bill the committee reported to the House on

March 29, 1965, had assumed a form which no one had predicted in the post-election certainty that some type of social security health insurance was forthcoming. The new bill included parts of the Administration bill, the Byrnes benefit package, and the AMA suggestion of an expanded Kerr-Mills program. These features were incorporated into two amendments to the Social Security Act: Title 18 and 19. Title 18's first section (Part A) included the hospital insurance program, the revised version of H.R. 1. Part B represented the modified Byrnes proposal of voluntary doctors' insurance. And Title 19 (now known as Medicaid) offered a liberalized Kerr-Mills program that, contrary to AMA intentions, was an addition to rather than a substitution for the other proposals. Essentially, the program provides for the unification of all medical vendor payments under state programs and uniform coverage for recipients. The provision in Title 19 which enables a state at its option to elect to cover individuals (regardless of age) not on public assistance, but whose incomes are close to the public assistance level, could also extend coverage to a significantly large portion of the poor population.

On the final vote of the committee, the Republicans held their ranks, and H.R. 6675 was reported out on a straight party vote of 17–8. When the House met on April 8 to vote on what had become known as the Mills bill, they gave the Ways and Means chairman a standing ovation. In a masterly explanation of the complicated measure (now 296 pages long), Mills demonstrated the thoroughness with which his committee had done its work. The health insurance program in H.R. 6675, Mills explained, was to cost about $3 billion. Byrnes presented his alternative bill after Mills had finished, and a vote was taken on whether to recommit H.R. 6675 in favor of the Republican alternative. The motion to recommit was defeated by 45 votes; 63 Democrats defected to the Republican measure, and only ten Republicans voted with the Democratic majority. Once it was clear that H.R. 6675 would pass, party lines re-formed and the House sent the Mills bill to the Senate by an overwhelming margin of 315–115.

What had changed Mills from a Medicare obstructionist to an

expansion-minded innovator? Critics speculated on whether the shift represented "rationality" or "rationalization," but none doubted Mills' central role in shaping the contents of the new legislative proposal. The puzzle includes two distinct issues: why did Mills seek to expand the Administration's bill, and what explains the form of the expansion he helped to engineer?

By changing from opponent to manager, Mills assured himself control of the content of H.R. 1 at a time when it could have been pushed through the Congress despite him. By encouraging innovation, and incorporating more generous benefits into the legislation, Mills undercut claims that his committee had produced an "inadequate" bill. In both respects, Mills became what Tom Wicker of *The New York Times* termed the "architect of victory for medical care, rather than just another devoted but defeated supporter" of the Kerr-Mills welfare approach *(New York Times,* 1965). Mills' conception of himself as the active head of an autonomous, technically expert committee helps explain his interest in shaping legislation he could no longer block, and his preoccupation with cautious financing of the social security system made him willing to combine benefit and financing arrangements that had been presented as mutually exclusive alternatives. The use of general revenues and beneficiary premiums in the financing of physicians' service insurance made certain the aged and the federal treasury, not the social security trust funds, would have to finance any benefit changes. In an interview during the summer of 1965, Mills explained that inclusion of medical insurance would "build a fence around the Medicare program" and forestall subsequent demands for liberalization that "might be a burden on the economy and the social security program." What Mills may have meant, as one government official explained off-the-record, was that Ways and Means could avoid "physician coverage in the future under social security by providing it now under the [Supplementary Medical Insurance] approach."

In sharp contrast to Mills' flexibility, HEW cautiously had settled for proposing its familiar King-Anderson plan. In comparison with the committed Medicare advocates, Mills was the more astute in realizing how much the Johnson landslide of 1964 had changed the constraints and incentives facing the 89th Congress. President Johnson, busy with the demands of a massive set of executive proposals, was willing to settle for the hospitalization insurance which the election had guaranteed. Liberal supporters of the Johnson Administration were astounded by Ways and Means' improvement of Medicare and befuddled by its causes. *The New Republic* (1965) captured the mood of this public at the time of the House vote, suggesting that the Mills bill could "only be discussed in superlatives":

> Fantastically enough, there was a tendency to expand [the Administration's bill] in the House Committee. Republicans and the American Medical Association complained that Medicare "did not go far enough." Trying to kill the bill they offered an alternative—a voluntary insurance plan covering doctor's fees, drugs, and similar services. What did the House Ways and Means Committee do? It added [these features] to its own bill. Will this pass? We don't know, but some bill will pass.

H.R. 6675 Passes the Senate: April-July

There was really no doubt that the expansion of Medicare would be sustained by the more liberal Senate and its Finance Committee. But the precise levels of benefits and form of administration were by no means certain. The Finance Committee Chairman, Russell Long (D., La.), held extended hearings during April and May, and the committee took nearly another month amending the House-passed bill in executive sessions. Two issues stood out in these discussions: whether to accept the payment method for in-hospital specialists on which Mills had insisted, and whether even more comprehensive benefits could be financed by varying the hospital deductible with the income of beneficiaries.

The first issue was taken up, with White House encouragement, by Senator Paul Douglas (D., Ill.). The question of specialist payment brought out in the open a dispute within the medical care industry. The American Hospital Association told the Finance Committee that encouraging hospital specialists to charge patients separately would both "tend to increase the overall cost of care to aged persons" and imperil the hospital as the "central institution in our health service system" (Feingold, 1966, 114). HEW's general counsel, Alanson Willcox, prepared a list of supporting arguments which Wilbur Cohen supplied in defense of the Douglas amendment to pay RAPP specialists as specified in the original H.R. 1. "These specialists," Willcox pointed out, "normally enjoy a monopoly of hospital business' and yet they seek the 'status of independent practitioners' without the burden of competition to which other practitioners are subject" (HEW 2, 1965).

The AMA responded with fury to Douglas' revisions. Defending the specialists, the AMA hailed Mills' payment plan as a way to break down the "corporate practice of medicine" which made radiologists, anaesthetics, pathologists, and physiatrists coerced "employees" of hospitals. "Medical care," the AMA told the Finance Committee, "is the responsibility of physicians, not hospitals" (Somers and Somers, 1967, 136). Apparently unconvinced, the Senators approved the Douglas amendment in early June.

In mid-June the Finance Committee approved a plan to eliminate time limits on the use of hospitals and nursing homes. The supporters of this amendment were a mixed lot of pro- and anti-Medicare Senators, and it was clear the latter group thought this change might deadlock the entire bill. For those who wanted more adequate protection against financial catastrophe there was the subsequent realization that a well-intentioned mistake had been made. With the White House and HEW insisting on a reconsideration, the committee scrapped the amendment on June 23 by a vote of 10–7. In its place, it provided "120 days of hospital care with $10 a day deductible after 60 days" (Wolkstein, 1968).

The Finance Committee also took up a variety of provisions within the Mills bill which Administration spokesmen considered "important defects." The Medicare sponsor in the Senate, Clinton Anderson, argued that paying physicians their "usual and custom-

ary fees" (the Byrnes suggestion) would "significantly and unneces-
sarily inflate the cost of the program to the tax-payer and to the
aged." The House bill had left the determination of what was a
"reasonable charge" to the insurance companies, which would act
as intermediaries for the medical insurance program, and Anderson
saw no reason why these companies would save the government
from an "open-ended payment" scheme (Bray, 1965). Medical
spokesmen, however, were so critical of the overall Medicare legislation that fears of a physicians' boycott persuaded Senate reformers not to raise further the sensitive topic of fee schedules for physicians.

The Senate, unlike the House, does not vote on social security
bills under a closed rule. This meant further amendments and debate would take place on the Senate floor on the Finance Committee's somewhat altered version of the Mills bill. On July 6 debate
was opened and the Senate quickly agreed to accept the recommendation to insure unlimited hospital care with $10 co-insurance pay-
ments after 60 days. Three days later, after heated discussion, the
Senate finished with its amendments, and passed its version of Medicare by a vote of 68–21. On the crucial but unsuccessful vote to
exclude Part A from the insurance program, 18 Republicans and 8
Southern Democrats took the losing side. According to newspaper
estimates, the expanded bill passed by the Senate increased the
"price tag on Medicare" by $900 million. The conference commit-
tee was certain to have a number of financial and administrative
differences to work out through compromise.

Medicare Comes out of the Conference Committee: July 26, 1965

More than 500 differences were resolved in conference between the
Senate and House versions of Medicare. Most of the changes were
made through the standard bargaining methods of *quid pro quo* and
splitting the difference. The most publicized decision was the rejection of the Douglas plan for paying RAPP specialists under the hospital insurance program. Mills' victory on this score was to cause

much further alarm in the months to come, when the Social Security Administration began its administrative task of preparing for Medicare's initiation, July 1, 1966.

The bulk of the decisions were compromises between divergent benefit levels. The changes of duration and type of benefit involved either accepting one of the two congressional versions or combining differing provisions. The decisions on the five basic benefits in the hospital plan aptly illustrate these patterns of accommodation:

1. *Benefit duration*—House provided 60 days of hospital care after a deductible of $40. Senate provided unlimited duration but with $10 co-insurance payments for each day in excess of 60. *Conference* provided 60 days with the $40 House deductible, and an additional 30 days with the Senate's $10 co-insurance provision.

2. *Posthospital extended care (skilled nursing home)*—House provided 20 days of such care with 2 additional days for each unused hospital day, but a maximum of 100 days. Senate provided 100 days but imposed a $5 a day co-insurance for each day in excess of 20. *Conference* adopted Senate version.

3. *Posthospital home-health visits*—House authorized 100 visits after hospitalization. Senate increased the number of visits to 175, and deleted requirements of hospitalization. *Conference* adopted House version.

4. *Outpatient diagnostic services*—House imposed a $20 deductible with this amount credited against an inaptient hospital deductible imposed at the same hospital within 20 days. Senate imposed a 20 percent co-insurance on such services, removed the credit against the inpatient hospital deductible but allowed a credit for the deductible as an incurred expense under the voluntary supplementary program (for deductible and reimbursement purposes). *Conference* adopted Senate version.

5. *Psychiatric facilities*—House provided for 60 days of hospital care with a 180-day lifetime limit in the voluntary supplemen-

tary program. Senate moved these services over into basic
hospital insurance and increased the lifetime limit to 210
days. *Conference* accepted the Senate version but reduced the
lifetime limit to 190 days *(Congressional Report* 3, 1965, 4).

None of these compromises satisfied the pro-Medicare pressure
groups which had been anxious to make the law administratively
less complicated. By late July, the conference committee had finished its report. On July 27, the House passed the revised bill by a
margin of 307–116 and the Senate followed suit two days later with
a 70–24 vote. On July 30, 1965, President Johnson signed the
Medicare bill into Public Law 89–97, at the ceremony in Independence, Missouri described at the beginning of this study.

The Outcome of 1965: Explanation and Issues

One of the most important lessons of Medicare's enactment is that
the events surrounding its passage were atypical. The massive Democratic electoral victories in 1964 created a solid majority in Congress for the President's social welfare bills, including federal aid to
education, Medicare, and the doubling of the "war on poverty" effort. To find the most recent precedent, we must go back almost 30
years, to Franklin Roosevelt's New Deal Congresses. In the inter-
vening years, we find a different pattern. Democratic majorities in
the Congress have not been uncommon, but normally the partisan
margins have been sufficiently close on many issues to give the balance of power to minority groups within the party. Under these circumstances, states' rights Southern congressmen in coalition with
Republicans have often been successful in blocking or delaying bills
which entail the expansion of federal control.

The fragmentation of authority in the Congress compounds the
opportunities for minorities to block legislation; bills must be subjected to committees, sub-committees, procedural formalities, and
conference groups. To be sure, overwhelming majority support for
a given bill can ensure that it will emerge, more or less intact, as

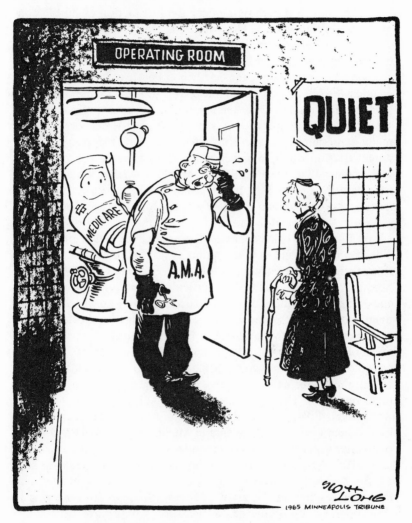

"THE OPERATION IS A FAILURE !...
THE PATIENT IS GOING TO LIVE!"

law, even though it may pass under the jurisdiction of hostile congressmen in the process. However, it is extraordinarily difficult to create a congressional majority committed to an issue out of Democratic congressional partisans. President Kennedy, in 1961, avoided a major confrontation over Medicare because it was uncertain whether the bill could pass a House vote and because he needed the support of Ways and Means members for his other programs. Congressmen must frequently make similar decisions; for example, many representatives who supported Medicare before 1965 were nonetheless unwilling to launch major drive to extract it from Ways and Means. Like the President, they often needed the support of Medicare opponents for other legislation which they believed was more important or had a better chance for successful enactment.

Within this context, backers of controversial legislation generally adopt a strategy which looks to the gradual accretion of support. They frame the issue so that opponents will find them difficult to attack, then set out to accumulate both mass public support and the necessary congressional votes. Particular attention is given to crucial committee bottlenecks. The Executive relies heavily on the influence of the House and Senate leadership in this effort, and acts on the assumption that although it is seldom possible to change the mind of a congressman on the merits of an issue, it is sometimes possible to change his vote. While the congressional leaders lack formal means for enforcing party discipline, they have a variety of other resources. Their personal influence with the regional caucuses who selected Ways and Means committeemen, for example, allowed them to deny assignments to Medicare opponents and thereby to alter gradually the voting margin on the committee.

By 1964, the use of this accretionist strategy by Medicare supporters seemed on the verge of success; and had the elections of that year resulted in the usual relatively close partisan margins in the Congress, the Medicare Act of 1965 would have been much narrower in scope, and its passage would stand as a vindication of the incrementalist strategy. In fact, the 1964 elections returned a

Congress in which many of the usual patterns of bargaining were less relevant. The Medicare bill which finally emerged as law must be analyzed in terms of the various responses to the highly unusual circumstances in that Congress.

In seeking answers as to why the legislative outcome differed so markedly from the Administration's input, three separable issues are involved. Why did the traditional hospitalization insurance proposal pass as one part of the composite legislation. The congressional realignment after the elections of 1964 provides the ready answer. Why the legislation took the composite form it did is partly answerable in this way as well. The certainty that some Medicare bill would be enacted changed the incentives and disincentives facing former Medicare opponents. Suggesting a physicians' insurance alternative offered an opportunity for Republicans to cut their losses in the face of certain Democratic victory and to counteract public identification of Republican opposition with intransigent AMA hostility to Medicare. Wilbur Mills' motives are fully comprehensible only in the context of congressional conventions especially the relationship of the Ways and Means Committee to the House, and the committee's tradition of restrained, consensual bargaining among its partisan blocs. However, if the political needs of the minority party and the Ways and Means members account for the Republican alternative bill and the committee's expansion of Medicare, the limits of that expansion require further explanation.

The context of the debate over government health insurance sharply delimited the range of alternatives open to innovators. That long debate—focused on the aged as the problem group, social security vs. general revenues as financing mechanisms, and partial vs. comprehensive benefits for either all the aged or only the very poor amongst the aged—structured the content of the innovations. The political circumstances of 1965 account for why innovation by Republicans and conservative Democrats was a sensible strategy. The character of more than a decade of dispute over health insurance programs for the aged explains the programmatic features of the combination that Wilbur Mills engineered, President Johnson took credit for, and the Republicans and American Medical Association inadvertently helped to ensure.

The outcome of 1965 was, to be sure, a model of unintended consequences. The final legislative package incorporated features which no one had fully foreseen, and aligned supporters and opponents in ways which surprised many of the leading actors. Yet the eleventh hour expansion of Medicare should not draw one's attention away from the constricting parameters of change. Were a European to reflect upon this episode of social policy making in America, his attention would be directed to the narrow range within which government health proposals operated. He would emphasize that no European nation restricted its health insurance programs to one age group; and he would point out that special health "assistance" programs, like that incorporated in Title 19, had been superceded in European countries for more than a generation. The European perspective is useful, if only to highlight those features of the 1965 Medicare legislation which were *not* changed.

Although the new law was broader than the King-Anderson bill in benefit structure, it did not provide payment for all medical expenses. P.L. 89–97 continued to reflect an "insurance" as opposed to a "prepayment" philosophy of medical-care financing. The former assumes that paying substantial portions of any insured cost is sufficient; the problem to which such a program addresses itself is avoidance of unbudgetable financial strain. The latter view seeks to separate financing from medical considerations. Its advocates are not satisfied with programs which pay 40 percent of the aged's expected medical expenses (one rough estimate of Medicare's effects); only full payment and the total removal of financial barriers to access to health services will satisfy them. In Medicare's range of deductibles, exclusions, and co-insurance provisions, the "insurance" approach was followed, illustrating the continuity between the first Ewing proposals in 1952 of 60 days of hospital care and the much-expanded benefits of the 1965 legislation.

Nor were major changes made in the group designated as beneficiaries under the insurance program. The Administration had single-mindedly focused on the aged and the legislation provided that "every person who has attained the age of 65" was entitled to hospital benefits. Though this coverage represented an expansion over the limitation to social security eligibles in bills of the 1950s and early 1960s, the legislation provided that, by 1968, the beneficiaries under Part A would be narrowed again to include only social security participants. (This provision "applied only to persons first attaining age 65 in 1968 and after—only a very small fraction of the current aged—and the test of social security eligibility is less strict than is the test for cash benefits" [Wolkstein, 1968].) The persistent efforts to provide Medicare benefits as a matter of "earned right" had prompted this focus on social security and, as a result, on the aged. While the social security system was not the only way to convey a sense of entitlement (payroll taxes in the Truman plans were included for the same purpose), the politics of more than a decade of incremental efforts had effectively undercut the broad coverage of the Truman proposals.

Title 19, establishing the medical assistance program popularly known as "Medicaid," made exception to the age restrictions. This bottom layer of the "legislative cake" authorized comprehensive coverage for all those, regardless of age, who qualified for public assistance and for those whose medical expenses threatened to produce future indigency. As in the Kerr-Mills bill which it succeeded, financing was to be shared by federal government general revenues and state funds. The Medicaid program, too, owed much to the past debates, growing as it did out of the welfare public assistance approach to social problems. Its attraction to the expansionists in 1965 did not rest on its charitable features alone. In the eyes of Wilbur Mills, it was yet another means of "building a fence" around Medicare, by undercutting future demands to expand the social security insurance program to cover all income groups.

The voluntary insurance scheme for physicians' services, Part B of Title 18, represented a return to the breadth of benefits suggested in the Truman plans (although, unlike the Truman proposals, it was neither compulsory nor available to all age groups). Since the adoption of an accretionist strategy in the wake of the Truman health insurance defeats, coverage of physicians' costs had been largely dropped from proposals. Throughout the 1950s reformers had focused on rising hospital costs and the role which the federal government should play in meeting those costs. Except for the For- and bills, proposals for health insurance between 1952 and 1964 fastidiously avoided the sensitive issue of covering doctors' care. Even when the election of 1964 eradicated the close congressional margin which had prompted the accretionist strategy in the first place, the Administration continued to follow it. It was Wilbur Mills, and not the presidential advisers, who most fully appreciated the changed possibilities. Once again acting to build a fence around the program and insure against later expansion of the social security program to include physicians' coverage, he pre-empted the Byrnes proposal with a general revenue-individual contribution payment scheme.

For a decade and more, the American Medical Association had been able to dictate many of the terms of debate, particularly on physicians' coverage. And although the 1964 election revealed how much the alleged power of AMA opposition to block legislation depended on the make-up of Congress, the provisions for paying doctors under Part B of Medicare reflected the legislators' fears that the doctors would act on their repeated threats of non-cooperation in implementing Medicare. To enlist the support of the medical profession, the law avoided prescribing a fee schedule for physicians, and directed instead that the doctors of Medicare patients be paid their "usual and customary fee," providing that the fee was also "reasonable." Moreover, it was not required that the doctor directly charge the insurance company intermediaries who were to handle the government payments; he could bill the patient, who, after paying his debt, would be reimbursed by the insurance company. This left a doctor the option of charging the patient more than the government would be willing to reimburse. But congressional sympathy with the doctors' distaste for government control, and fear that doctors would elect not to treat Medicare patients under more restrictive fee schedules, made "reasonable charges" appear a sensible standard of payment.

The eligibility requirements, benefits, and financing of the Medicare program represent a complex political outcome, a mixture of continuity and surprise not typical of the legislative histories of other social welfare measures. The long process of building support for a hospitalization program covering the aged had not prepared the Johnson Administration for the unpredictable opportunities of 1965. Instead of the King-Anderson bills of the 1960s, HEW had the Mills bill to turn into an operational Medicare program by July, 1966. The politics of congressional bargaining had produced a considerably larger (and many felt a better) bill than the Johnson Administration had proposed in the first weeks of 1965.

5

Epilogue

The Medicare program has been in effect since July 1, 1966. In the year which intervened between enactment and the first payment of benefits, the Social Security Administration involved itself in massive preparatory tasks. The most important of these was to contact the aged and inform them of their rights to coverage and benefits under the program. Enrollment of the aged in the voluntary medical insurance program, Part B of Title 18, posed the greatest publicity problem. Aged citizens were required to sign up and begin payment of the $3 monthly premiums in order to participate. Since the success of this Supplementary Medical Insurance Program depended on voluntary enrollment, the Social Security Administration launched an intensive promotional campaign in local and national news media, aimed at encouraging the aged to participate. More than half of the 50 states took the initiative in enrolling and assuming the premium payments for those amongst the aged who were on the state public assistance rolls. At the end of the first year of Medicare's operation, the success of the recruitment program was evident:

—of the approximately 19 million aged citizens, 93 percent, or 17.7 million, were enrolled in the voluntary medical insurance program (Part B of Title 18).

—one in five of America's elderly had entered a hospital under the new law, and twelve million had used Part B services.

—hospital expenses accounted for $2.5 billion of the $3.2 billion expended by the SSA for Medicare.

—on the average, patients were reimbursed for 80 percent of their hospital expenses, and Medicare covered $600 of the $750 average bill (HEW 2, 1967).

In addition to enrolling potential patients, the Social Security Administration was given the task of evaluating health facilities, i.e., hospitals, nursing homes and home health agencies. The Medicare law required that health facilities apply to participate and meet several conditions specified in the law before they could receive reimbursement for services provided to Medicare patients. Besides satisfying several standards designed to ensure a higher quality of care, the institution had to offer proof that its services were rendered on a non-discriminatory basis, in compliance with the Civil Rights Act of 1964. These requirements frequently posed difficulties for the Medicare administrators. In many cases, hospitals which were unable or unwilling to meet the certification standards were also the only facilities available to Medicare patients in their localities. On the eve of Medicare's initiation, the non-discriminatory requirement was embroiling the government in a well-publicized confrontation with some Southern hospitals who were willing to risk exclusion from the Medicare program before desegregating their facilities. Civil rights lawyers saw Medicare as a powerful instrument for change. But the price of change was the willingness to deny (in extreme cases of non-compliance) Medicare benefits to aged persons who happened to live in areas of segregation. This dilemma has by no means been resolved. But it is certain that there were hospitals in

the South receiving Medicare benefits whose facilities were still substantially segregated (Schecter, 1968).

The first year of operation brought a mixture of problems and ful-
filment. The worst fears that Medicare patients would crowd the
hospitals beyond their capacity were nowhere realized. Some physicians refused to cooperate, but the AMA president, Dr. James Ap-
pel, was successful in directing his organization's energies away
from threats of boycotts to consultations about the terms of medical
service. At the same time, the Administration was pleased with the
high utilization rates under the program.

The problems in administering Medicare arose not so much in
connection with earlier fears as with issues that had not been widely
raised at the time of passage. Some of the administrative problems
were typical of large new governmental programs and hence predictable. There were delays in paying providers of service, particularly during the first summer of operations. The fact that such delay
was not surprising hardly allayed the irritation of the hospitals,
nursing homes, and doctors affected.

The most serious and persistent of the problems concerned the
methods and costs of paying doctors and hospitals under Medicare.
The statute had purposely avoided setting a specific limit on the
amount a doctor could charge a Medicare patient, and specified instead that physicians were to be paid "reasonable charges." The
lawmakers assumed that such charges would be higher than those
customarily charged low-income patients, lest Medicare patients be
treated as charity cases. The "reasonable charge" was defined as
one which was "customary" for the individual physician, and no
higher than the charges "prevailing" in his locale or those regularly
paid by the insurance intermediary in comparable circumstances.
(The use of insurance companies as decentralized payment administrators was another surprise of the legislative politics.) For all its
seeming clarity, this standard was unworkable in the context of
Medicare's first year. No one knew what doctors were customarily
charging. There was no agreement among doctors or government
officials about what constituted the upper limit of "prevailing

charges." And, although Blue Shield and commercial insurance comapnies had evidence about their own past payments, there was no agreement about what constituted "comparable services" in "comparable circumstances." Medicare thus began with an open-ended payment method for physicians. Doctors were as uncertain as everyone else about how the law would be construed, and fears that the insurance intermediaries would codify and freeze their definitions of "reasonable charges" gave physicians every incentive to raise their fees (Marmor, 1968). In the year between enactment of the Medicare law and its initial operation, the rate of increase in physician fees more than doubled (see table 1).

TABLE 1—Increase in Physicians' Fees

	1964	1965	1966	1967
Physician Fee Index	2.4%	3.8%	7.8%	6.1%
Consumer Price Index	1.3	2.0	3.3	3.1

Some portion of that increase was caused by Medicare's payment method, and the continuing overall rise in physician fees has presented serious political problems.

Hospital price increases presented the most intractable political problem for the Johnson Administration. In the first year of Medicare's operation, the average daily service charge in America's hospitals increased by an unprecedented 21.9 percent (chart 3). Each month the Labor Department's consumer price survey reported further increases, and by the summer of 1967 President Johnson asked HEW Secretary John Gardner to "study the reasons behind the rapid rise in the price of medical care and to offer recommendations for moderating that rise." Five months later Gardiner reported that the Medicare program, by requiring hospitals to re-examine their costs and charges, had probably prompted many hospitals "to increase their charges" (HEW 3, 1967). The HEW report concluded that the question for the future "is not whether medical prices will rise, but how fast they will rise." This problem, accentuated but not caused alone by the Medicare program, would remain a worri-

CHART 3

Quarterly Index of Consumer and Medical Care Prices, 1959–67

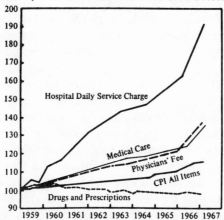

SOURCE: Dorothy P. Rice and Barbara S. Cooper, "National Health Expenditures, 1950–66," U.S. Department of Health, Education, and Welfare, *Social Security Bulletin,* April, 1968, p. 12.

some political issue. In the State of the Union Address, January 17, 1968, President Johnson illustrated how the government's expanded role in financing personal health services had enlarged its responsibility for controlling price increases; measures would be proposed, the President promised, to "stem the rising costs of medical care." While hospital costs have continued to rise faster than other components of the medical care price index, the rate of increase decelerated sharply in the second year of the Medicare program from 21.9 percent in the June 1966–June 1967 period to 12.2 percent in the following year (Rice and Horowitz, 1968).

The disputes over the causes and consequences of medical price increases revealed in a striking way the differences between the politics of legislation and those of administration. Once Medicare was enacted, its publicity value dropped sharply. The press no longer had the drama of committee clashes or heated congressional debates to report to their audiences. The broad alignment of opposing economic interests that had marked the earlier Medicare debate fell

apart as the issue turned from whether the government would insure the aged against health expenses to how it would do so.
Groups in the medical care industry remained active, but their activities were consultative and relatively unpublicized, not those of
diehard ideological adversaries. Administrative lobbyists representing hospitals, physicians, nurses, and nursing homes continually
pressed their claims on the Social Security Administration and
through their trade journals kept members aware of the actual
workings of the Medicare program. In the process, the voice of the
consumer became less distinct. The claims of the aged consumer
are less salient symbolic issues than those of elderly persons pressing for the statutory redistribution of medical care. Congressmen
passed on the complaints of their aged constituents, and in the case
of hardships caused by the program's regulations for reimbursing
physicians who directly billed their patients, there was ameliorative
legislative action in 1967. Although a bill to include the disabled
under Medicare provisions was defeated in 1967, no one in the
Johnson Administration pressed for massive extensions of the program. (More recently, however, the unabated rise in medical care
prices seems to be stimulating revived interest in universal health
insurance. In 1968, a labor-supported Committee for National
Health Insurance was organized, and in summer of 1969, the
American Hospital Association announced that it was studying the
feasibility of a national health insurance plan in the United States.)
    One of the fascinating features of the Medicare story has been
the succession of new issues, unexpected outcomes, and surprising
conjunctions of events. In two decades of debate about government
health insurance, almost no one pressed the issue of racially segregated medical services. Yet in the first weeks of the program, the
question of certifying Southern hospitals under Medicare took up
more of the time of HEW's three top health officials than any other
feature of the Medicare program. The methods of paying physicians
and hospitals were among the most intractable issues facing the Social Security administrators. Yet for years no one had imagined
paying physicians under a Medicare program and no office of the

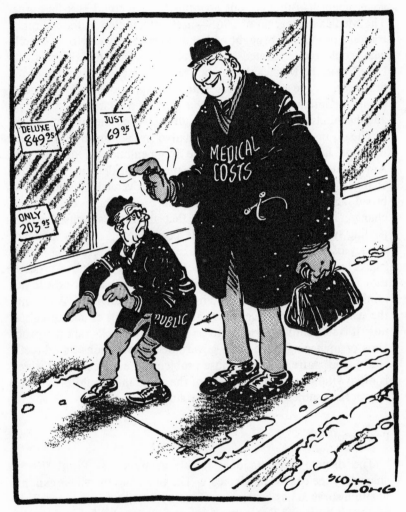

"SICK OF INFLATION? BUSTER, YOU DON'T DARE GET SICK!"

government had thought out how this burden could best be borne. The Medicaid program of 1965—itself an addition to the Administration's proposal—brought with it serious controversy over exactly who would be designated as medically indigent. In California and New York, the Medicaid program faced financial difficulties in the first year, as the price increases and unexpectedly high utilization strained administrative budgets and prompted charges that doctors and hospitals were taking unfair advantage of the new program.

The disjunction between the legislative and administrative politics was not, however, surprising. The fragmentation of authority in American politics, the myriad opportunities for delaying legislative change—both entail that promoters of controversial legislation seek broad agreement among a wide variety of publics on minimal change. The consequence of this is that attention is focused on appealing symbols and slogans: the desperation of the aged, the inadequacy of private insurance coverage, the fear of 'creeping socialism.' However crucial these disputes are for the legislative process, they provide no answers (indeed little discussion) about how to administer a program whose enactment was once divisive. And, with the usual American uncertainty about the timing of social legislation, it is not until programs are on the statute books that the problems of managing large-scale government innovations are directly confronted. A treatment of those problems, the resolution of which is often vital to the effectiveness of the program, would provide an appropriate subject for another case study.

Postscript

The dispute over national health insurance in the 1970s is shaped by the origins of Medicare. The processes by which national health insurance has become a salient U. S. political issue recall the Medicare episode. The contestants remain markedly similar, and the contest raises similar issues of public vs. private control, cost and price increases, federalism, and the like. Moreover, within the government, the same departments and committees involved in Medicare will deal with national health insurance.

TABLE 2—Total and Per Capita Hospital and Medical Insurance Expenditures, Fiscal Years 1967–71

Program	Fiscal year				
	1967	1968	1969	1970	1971
	Amount (in millions)				
Hospital and medical insurance	$3,395	$5,347	$6,598	$7,149	$7,875
Benefit payments	3,172	5,126	6,299	6,784	7,478
Administrative expenses	223	221	299	366	397
Hospital insurance	2,597	3,815	4,757	4,953	5,592
Benefit payments	2,508	3,736	4,654	4,804	5,443
Administrative expenses	89	79	104	149	149
Medical insurance	798	1,532	1,840	2,196	2,283
Benefit payments	664	1,390	1,645	1,979	2,035
Administrative expenses	134	143	195	217	248
	Per capita amount				
Hospital and medical insurance	$178	$274	$333	$353	$380
Benefit payments	166	263	318	335	361
Administrative expenses	12	11	15	18	19
Hospital insurance	136	196	241	246	272
Benefit payments	131	192	236	238	265
Administrative expenses	5	4	5	7	7
Medical insurance	45	85	98	114	116
Benefit payments	37	77	87	102	103
Administrative expenses	8	8	10	11	13
	Percentage change from preceding fiscal year				
Hospital and medical insurance		57.5	23.4	8.4	10.2
Benefit payments		61.6	22.9	7.7	10.2
Administrative expenses		−.6	35.1	22.4	8.6
Hospital insurance		46.9	24.7	4.1	12.9
Benefit payments		49.0	24.6	3.2	13.3
Administrative expenses		−11.5	32.5	42.7	.6
Medical insurance		92.0	20.1	19.4	3.9
Benefit payments		109.2	18.4	20.3	2.8
Administrative expenses		6.7	36.5	11.5	14.1

SOURCE: Howard West, "Five Years of Medicare—A Statistical Review," *Social Security Bulletin*, Dec. 1971, p. 20.

TABLE 3—Annual Percentage Changes in Physician Fees According to the Consumer Price Index for the Fiscal Years 1967–71.

Fiscal year	Physicians' fees (index, calendar year 1967=100)	Percentage increase
1967	96.9	7.4
1968	102.8	6.1
1969	109.1	6.1
1970	117.0	7.2
1971	125.8	7.5

SOURCE: Howard West, "Five Years of Medicare—A Statistical Review," *Social Security Bulletin*, Dec. 1971, p. 21.

TABLE 4—Consumer Price Index and American Hospital Association Data for Hospital Expenses, Each Fiscal Year, 1967–71, and Annual Percentage Increases

Fiscal year	Hospital daily service charges		Hospital expenses per patient day (AHA)	
	Index (calendar year 1967=100)	Annual percentage increase	Amount	Annual percentage increase
1967	92.2	16.6	$53.67	12.5
1968	106.4	15.4	61.73	15.0
1969	120.5	13.3	70.13	13.6
1970	135.4	12.4	80.71	15.1
1971	152.8	12.9	91.37	13.2

SOURCE: Data for daily service charges are from the *Consumer Price Index*, Bureau of Labor Statistics; data for hospital expenses per patient day are from "Hospital Indicators," *Hospitals*, Journal of the American Hospital Association. (From Howard West, "Five Years of Medicare—A Statistical Review." *Social Security Bulletin*, Dec. 1971, p. 21.

Similar developments do not of course mean identical ones. The experience with Medicare and Medicaid in the late 1960s occasioned the discussion of national health insurance and shaped its character in ways without precedent in the Medicare case. After five years of experience with these programs, there is widespread anxiety about the adequacy and financing of our health-care system. In part, the anxiety is over increased government expenditures for health care amounting in 1971 to nearly $14 billion for Medicare and Medicaid alone. Table 2 makes plain the rapid increases of expenditures for Medicare over its first five years.

The inflation of physicians' fees and hospital daily service charges have also become symbols of a health-care crisis. The relatively high annual rates of increase for both items are set out in tables 3 and 4 for the 1967–71 period.

The increases in the cost of medical care will become the central problem focus in the debate over national health insurance. But just as with the plight of the aged in the fight over Medicare, the agreement about a cost crisis will not produce concensus about its cures or consequences. Nonetheless, those interested in public choice over U. S. health insurance might well find the account of Medicare policy-making relevant to their concerns.

6

Medicare and the Analysis of Social Policy in American Politics

Case Studies and Cumulative Knowledge

Case studies cannot by their nature prove anything. They can only illustrate the plausibility (or implausibility) of other conceptual, procedural, or substantive generalizations. This final chapter departs from the sequential organization of the earlier part of the book to explore the significance of the Medicare case and to attempt to set out some of these other evaluations. First, I discuss the underlying framework of analysis which guided the way I posed and tried to answer my inquiries. My interest in analytic frameworks arises from a concern that case studies be more cumulative than they have been. Only studies that employ comparable analytic models can be cumulated, and the first part of this chapter discusses both some representative analytic models and the use put to them in the bulk of the Medicare analysis.

Second, I compare the political processes and policy outcomes of Medicare with those of other issues to show how the processes that characterized the Medicare dispute are general to the redistributive arena of American politics. In policy content, Medicare exemplifies the social insurance model of welfare policy. Its beneficiaries, benefits, financing, and administrative structure conform strikingly to this pattern and are in equally striking contrast with those of public assistance programs.

Third, this concluding chapter addresses itself to some of the differences between legislative and administrative politics. The early implementation of Medicare illustrates the transformation of controversial, statutory proposals into operational programs which quickly become routinized, stripped of earlier ideological conflict, and beset by the competing and intense claims of groups materially concerned with their burdens and benefits.

Conceptual Models and the Medicare Case

The discussion of Medicare politics earlier in this book was organized with self-conscious concern about how its conceptual structure could be adapted to cumulative policy analysis. This meant a continuing concern with how the problems of analysis were framed, what units of analysis were used, what focal concepts, and what patterns of inference. I want to make these underlying concerns explicit at this point and consider the explanatory effects of alternative analytic frameworks.

Conceptual frameworks give structure to the complex political universe for the analyst and in that sense are like lenses, that is, instruments that shape the field of vision, determine the level of detail, color the objects viewed, and limit the range of consideration. In reviewing the Medicare analysis from this standpoint, one is led to ask, "What framework was implicit in its various parts, and what difference did it make in the analysis offered?"

The Origins of Medicare: The Rational Actor Model

In dealing with the origins of Medicare, the question was why government elites *chose* in the early 1950s to narrow the focus of federal health insurance bills from the general population to the aged, and to restrict benefits to partial hospitalization coverage. Why, in short, did the Truman Administration decide to adopt the Medicare strategy?

The unit of analysis used in the text was a strategic political decision. The explanation given for the strategic choice was in the form of a set of reasons why sensible men could agree on a new but less dramatic course of action. This type of explanation should be distinguished from an account of why the shift in strategy took place. Useless debate is furthered without care for such distinctions. The reasons men give for a course of action may differ widely from the fundamental causes for a course of action—in this case, a shift in political strategy.

The fate of the Truman health insurance proposals provided the immediate backdrop for strategic choice. The perception that the aged were more acceptable to the general public as a deserving group was the major reason they were the chosen target of concern. Likewise, the restriction of Medicare benefits to social security beneficiaries was explained by the observation that social insurance programs enjoy considerable legitimacy while public assistance programs that use the means test do not. The principal pattern of inference was to show what goals the reformers were pursuing in deciding to opt for the Medicare rather than the national health insurance strategy.

Thinking about a government as if it were a single rational actor is perhaps the most common analytic orientation of U. S. political scientists. The vocabulary of "choice," "purposive action," and "rational calculation" is so common in national policy studies that its users are not typically self-conscious about the assumptions on which their conceptual orientation depends. For many purposes, political occurrences may be properly characterized as the purposive acts of national governments, to summarize the varied activities of governmental representatives as the nation transforms "unwieldy complexity into manageable packages" (Allison, 1968, 1). But this productive shorthand has the capacity to obscure as well as aid; it does not take into account that what we call the government is in fact a loose congerie of large organizations and political bargainers.

According to the rational actor model, the happenings of national politics are "the choices of domestic actors." Policy is understood as the action of the rational decision-maker. The choices and actions of the nation are thus "viewed as means calculated to achieve national goals and purposes." Such actions are interpreted as solutions to domestic problems such that the "explanation of rational action consists of showing what goal the nation was pursuing in committing the action and how in the light of that goal the action was the most reasonable choice." The implication is that important policy decisions have big causes, that large organizations perform important actions to serve substantial purposes. Analysts employing this framework may disagree sharply on which causes, which reasons, and which purposes are associated with particular governmental decisions, but the similarity of their purposive analytic orientation is striking (Allison, 1968, 1 ff.).

The basic unit of analysis in such work is the government's choice of strategy. The central concepts include the government as actor, governmental goals, alternative solutions, calculation, and consequences. These characteristic concepts are employed in a distinctive pattern of inference.

As Allison suggests, "if a nation or state or city has specific objectives, it will choose the optimal means towards those objectives." Conversely, if the "nation chooses an action or makes a decision, its goals can be inferred by calculating what are the ends towards which those acts constitute optimum means" (1968, 9). The result is a type of explanatory logic in which the knowledge of either goals or actions leads to an explanation of the other. Portraying governments as rational actors thus involves a characteristic model of description, explanation, and (one could show) prediction and evaluation.

Had the question of Medicare's origins been raised in organizational or bargaining terms, both the formulation and solution of the puzzle would have been different. From an organizational perspective, the question of Medicare's origins would have focused on the process by which health insurance for the aged arose as a political issue. Such an analysis would have characterized the relevant organizational units concerned with health and the aged, their standard ways of receiving, generating, and interpreting information, and their ordinary rules of decision for political strategy. Also, chapter 1 would have dealt extensively with the organizational setting of the Medicare strategy; the central issue would have been "How is it that the shift in health insurance strategy took place?" The relevant answer would have been not so much reasons why that decision made sense but rather why those reasons made sense to the organizational actors and how that led them to take this different posture toward the problems and possibilities of health insurance in American politics. Organizational analysis would emphasize that information on the aged was more readily available to organizations like the Federal Security Agency, a group charged with responsibility for the aged generally, and social security beneficiaries particularly. The reasons for concentrating on the aged would, from this view, be very different from the reasons why the aged warranted, in an objective analysis, special health concern.

My purpose here is not to treat alternative analytic frameworks as mutually exclusive. They are less discrete than that, and the analysis of a topic like Medicare's origins inevitably mixes elements of a number of analytic approaches. But I do want to emphasize the focus of attention in chapter 1. It was on the decision to adopt a Medicare strategy and differed from the organizational analyst's interest in how a particular set of complex events takes place. Students of bureaucratic bargaining would have raised still different questions about Medicare's origins as a public issue. They would treat the Medicare strategy decision as part of an ongoing policy contest in which the most stubborn advocates of the Truman health proposals were defeated by the proponents of incrementalism. Detailed information about the actors involved and the governmental atmosphere in which the Ewing plan emerged would be required for this type of analysis. Very little appears in this book about the structure of the Federal Security Agency, its relations with the Truman staff, and its connections with congressional health insurance advocates.

It is precisely that sort of evidence which permits characterizing a bargaining game out of which a strategic choice emerges. Such a view not only stresses political victors and losers, but treats decisions as part of an ongoing struggle. The shift to a Medicare approach is but one stage in a fluid policy development; the incentives of key actors to promote or oppose this shift would be part of an overall portrait of the health-politics field. Some of this perspective was evident in the detail included in chapter 1. The prominent position within the Federal Security Agency of such long-time social security experts as Wilbur Cohen and I. S. Falk helped to explain the availability of a social insurance alternative to the Truman plan. (It should be remembered that both these officials were advocates of general health insurance, but less sanguine than others as to its political feasibility.) The access Cohen and Falk had to Oscar Ewing constituted a crucial bargaining advantage for those seeking a limited, but more politically appealing health insurance initiative. The difference between explaining why health insurance for the aged made sense and why that decision was adopted should by now be more apparent. In chapter 1 we permitted the answer to the former question to serve as a parsimonious proxy for the latter.

The Responses of Medicare, 1952-64: The Organizational Process Model

The second topic of this book is the fate of Medicare proposals *after* the Ewing-Truman decision. We were interested in the contestants about Medicare and the nature of the contest over time. Here our concern for describing and accounting for a *pattern* of organizational behavior makes the rational actor framework less useful. The immediate organizational problems of concerned pressure groups at this point took precedence over the social problems of the aged to which the advocates of Medicare had drawn attention. In discussing this aspect of the problem, we were less interested in Medicare as a rational response to the problems of the elderly and more concerned with the use made of their woes by pressure group antagonists. In characterizing the Medicare contest, we concentrated on the major organizational units concerned and, implicitly, employed some of the characteristic features of what has been called the organizational process model (Allison, 1968, 3).

According to the organizational process model, what the rational policy analysts calls *choices* and *acts* are in fact outputs of organizations functioning according to standard patterns of behavior. To explain a particular occurrence, one "identifies the relevant organization" (or organizations) and "displays the pattern of procedures and conventions out of which the action emerged." The basic unit of analysis is the organization, and the focal concepts include routine behavior, standard operating procedures, biased information, incremental change, and organizational perspective (Allison, 1968, 3).

Explanations in organizational terms typically "focus on the pattern of statements, directives, and actions of relevant agencies and departments." A central assumption is that organizations change slowly, that behavior in time $t + 1$ will resemble that of time t. Predictions thus are based on the "structure, programs, and past behavior of the relevant organizations" (Allison, 1968, 22). Throughout, our central concern is how certain patterns of activity take place in the special organizations we call government.

Chapters 2 and 3 stress that both the contest and the contestants over Medicare remained remarkably stable in the period 1952–64, "two well-defined camps with opposing views, camps with few individuals who were impartial or uncommitted" (c.f. Wildavsky, 1962, 304). The breadth of the conflict over Medicare was illustrated by the large number of concerned groups (often otherwise not involved with health issues) and their ideological polarization. The disputes over Medicare had recurring, predictable features even as the specific proposals in question changed substantially. The disputants—like adversaries in open class conflict—called upon crystallized attitudes and positions and expressed them in distinctive ways to identify problems and frame remedies. The stability in Medicare demands and reactions permitted a relatively static description of group conflict on this issue.

The stereotypical and static quality of the fight over Medicare is more readily understandable when one considers the size and character of the parties to it.* Large national associations like the AMA and AFL-CIO have widely dispersed component parts; they function in part as Washington lobbyists for issues affecting the interests of widely disparate members. Hence, they must seek common denominators of sentiment that will satisfy the organization's leading actors without antagonizing large bodies of more passive members. Such large organizations are specialized, with full-time staffs devoted to preparing responses to public policy questions when the occasion arises and in the direction dictated by past organizational attitudes. These attitudes are slow to change and help account for the predictable way in which sides were taken on various Medicare proposals over time. Intelligence and research were weapons in a long struggle between groups that distrusted each other. Hence, it is not surprising that the debate was stable; mutually incompatible positions on health insurance arose in part from the maintenance needs of large-scale organizations (and their leaders).

An organizational perspective was appropriate for analyzing the *pattern* of Medicare debates and debaters. In dealing with that pattern it was useful to concentrate on the predictable behavior of the large pressure groups involved. Students of organizations know that such collectivities do not behave like individuals. Organizations filter information in ways persons do not. They seek means to main-

---

* It might be objected that stereotypes and simplified images of opponents are characteristic of most political disputes. But any one who has, for example, surveyed the hearings of regulatory bodies will recognize an attention to evidential canons never present when Medicare antagonists aired their views, whether in the press or during congressional hearings. Part of the reason, of course, is that Medicare actors were directing their remarks to a much wider audience and naturally relied on compelling symbols where complex factual presentations would have been confusing or boring.

tain themselves over time not characteristic of individual behavior. The conjunction of the routine behavior of many individuals in organizational settings has results in public policy for which one cannot account by looking only at the activities of isolated individuals.

Other questions could have been raised about the long fight over Medicare. Had one concentrated on explaining a particular response to a particular proposal (the 1961 congressional battle, for instance), it would have been more appropriate to stress individual actions and the individual bargaining that characterized that episode. That was precisely the approach used in discussing 1961 events, and, in particular, the 1965 legislative outcome.

The 1965 Legislation: The Bureaucratic Politics Model

The enactment of Medicare was treated in earlier chapters primarily as the result of a bargaining game in which none of the rele- vant executive, legislative, or pressure-group players could fully control the outcome. The key actors—Mills and Byrnes of the Ways and Means Committee, Cohen of HEW, Long and Anderson of the Senate Finance Committee, the AMA and the labor leaders —all had different conceptions of the problem at hand. They had different stakes in the outcome of the legislative struggle and different terms on which they were willing to compromise.

Not only was bargaining stressed—both explicit and tacit—but also the decentralized nature of the American political process. It was never clear at what stage in the legislative process major alterations were or were not possible. The statutory result could not be interpreted solely as the product of the Administration's intentions. Rather, it emerged as the outcome of a long, complicated struggle and the law in its final form was not one which any of the major actors intended at the outset.

The bureaucratic politics framework considers "domestic policy to consist of *outcomes* of a series of overlapping bargaining games" arranged heirarchically within the national government. Two descriptive emphases are involved: that governments are made up of

disparate, decentralized organizations headed by leaders with unequal power, and that such leaders, in the course of policy-making,
engage in bargaining. These players, operating with different
perspectives and different priorities, struggle for preferred outcomes with the power at their disposal. Explanations in this third
model proceed from descriptions of the "position and power of the
principal players" and concentrate on the "understandings and misunderstandings which determine the outcome of the game" (Allison, 1968, 3).

The basic unit of analysis is the decentralized bargaining game
played by relatively autonomous actors. The focal concepts include
bargaining strategies, roles, moves, stakes, trade-offs, tactics, and
conventions (or rules of the game). Explanations that employ this
framework typically draw upon the stakes and interests the actors
bring to disputes about particular policy issues. The decisions and
actions of governments constitute outcomes in the "sense that what
happens is not chosen as a solution to a problem" but is rather the
result of "political bargaining among a number of independent
players, of compromise, coalition, competition, and confusion
among government officials many of whom are focusing on different faces of the issue." The actions of government—the sum of the
"behavior of representatives of a government" involved in a policy
issue—"is rarely intended by any individual or group." From this
characterization of policy-making come distinctive patterns of inference, rules of explanation such as "where you stand depends on
where you sit." Moreover, important government decisions are not
viewed as the result of a single game. Rather, what the government
does is a "collage of individual acts, outcomes of minor and major
games, and foul-ups." The understanding of that cumulative process requires piece-by-piece disaggregation of the policy-making.
What moves the process, in any event, is not simply the "reasons
which support a course of action, nor the routines of organizations
which enact an alternative, but the power and skill of proponents
and opponents of the action in question" (Allison, 1968, 26 ff.).

Treating statutes as bargaining outcomes requires the sort of detailed characterization of individual styles, interests, and position which chapter 4 presented. Actors like Mills, for instance, no longer asked in January, 1965, whether it was preferable that the U.S. Government provide hospital and nursing home insurance for the aged under social security. That much was a foregone conclusion which shaped the behavior of an adaptive committee chairman like Mills. He could in 1965 be a reluctant bystander or an adroit manager of legislation which in another setting he would have preferred to block. Mills has always adjusted to legislative certainty and tried to take charge of the form which the inevitable takes. Cutting back on the Administration's proposal in 1965 was an extraordinarily difficult alternative, given that the problems of the aged had been identified in a way for which the "input" of H.R. 1 was at best a partial solution. Moreover, scrimping on the aged when legislation was imminent was more difficult than preventing any Medicare action whatsoever in the period before 1965. These were the types of considerations which dominated the presentation of chapter 4: evidence about the rules of the legislative game, the stakes involved, and the radically altered nature of the 1965 setting. The bargaining which took place should not be allowed to obscure the vital fact that the election of 1964 had given all the actors less to bargain about.

We have thus far concentrated on showing how different analytic approaches lead to distinguishable sets of questions about public policy developments like Medicare legislation. It should be added that they also make a difference in the evaluations, recommendations, and predictions one makes about public policy. Consider some of the predictive and prescriptive differences that would emerge from alternative approaches to the explanation of the Medicare statute. The analyst who viewed Medicare legislation as the national solution to a pressing social problem would expect (and predict) that periodic adjustments would be made to make the program a more efficient instrument to cope with the health and financial problems of the aged. He would expect monitoring of the program as part of the effort to increase the level of achievement of the original national goal.*

Contrast these predictions with those a bargaining analyst would make on the basis of chapter 4. He would expect future outcomes to vary with what one might call the deal of the electoral cards. Since the innovations of 1965 were so much the result of the atypical partisan makeup of the 88th Congress, he would predict less innovation in more typical Congresses. He would not expect the Committee on Ways and Means, for instance, to preoccupy itself with improving the program, or to seek aggressively alternative means to meet the health needs of other Americans not assisted by Medicare.

Political recommendations would be equally different. One could imagine problem-solvers trying to convince the congressional committee that new difficulties, such as higher medical prices, have arisen for the aged, or that more serious health and financial problems are being felt by the disadvantaged and poor. The emphasis here would be on identifying the social ills for which national action is required. Students of bargaining would offer different recommendations. They would stress continued efforts to reshape the Committee on Ways and Means, taking cues from the "packing" of the committee after 1961. They would advise political investments of this kind, rather than a search for problems, as the best means of insuring action on health problems we are already well aware of. Viewed from the anti-Medicare perspective, bargaining students would firmly recommend prevention of these long-term investments. These illustrations—admittedly brief and elliptical—are examples of the differences which analytic lenses may make in what we see, predict, and recommend about public policy.

---

* This follows from the assumption that the problem was financial inability of the aged to manage their health costs. If the "problem" had been defined as coping with the demand by unions, the aged, and others for "some" health care assistance, the legislation of 1965 might well be considered a rational (and nearly complete) solution.

Processes and Policy in American Politics: The Case of Medicare

The preceding analytic discussion raised issues about studying American public policy that were not explicitly discussed in the case study itself. In turning to the relation between Medicare politics and more general characterizations of American political life, I will try to make systematic the observations and connections that were intermittently raised in the first five chapters. There is a substantial literature on American political processes and considerable evidence of what is taken to be distinctive about the politics of some subject matter (tariffs or housing) or some broad class of policies (regulatory or distributive). The first part of the following discussion will compare Medicare findings with these broader generalizations; its aim is to present evidence why some generalizations appear plausible, though, by its nature, case study material cannot constitute a definitive test. The second part will compare the substance of Medicare policy with other views of the typical allocative and redistributive policies generated in American politics.

Political scientists have expended great efforts in recent years trying to specify the ways by which different issues are raised, disputed, coped with, and sometimes "solved." Lowi (1964) has provided a typology for discriminating among public policies which usefully categorizes the Medicare case. He describes three major patterns of political conflict which are said to be associated with three different types of public policies—*distributive, regulative,* and *redistributive.* Distributive policies, which parcel out public benefits to interested parties, provoke a stable alliance of diverse groups that seek portions of the pork barrel. Regulative policies, which constrain the relations among competing groups and persons, provide incentives for shifting coalitions, pluralistic competition, and the standard forms of compromise. Redistributive policies, which reallocate benefits and burdens among broad socioeconomic population groups, foster polarized and enduring conflict in which large national pressure groups play central roles.

Lowi characterizes three patterns of conflict, but identifies them by their putative cause—the type of policy.* It is clear that actual policies are never so distinct. All public programs redistribute resources, but most are not primarily attempts to do so. Likewise, all government programs depend upon an ultimate capacity to regulate the conduct of citizens, but most do not make such regulation their prime object. And almost all government programs involve the distribution of goods and services among different groups, though the question of which county or which social class should receive them is not always salient. But whatever the cause of the pattern of conflict, one can assess which pattern is illustrated by individual policy conflicts like Medicare.

The conflict over Medicare mirrors the political processes Lowi identifies with "redistributive" policies. The themes of that conflict —the threat of "big government," the interests of the have-nots vs. the haves—illustrate the cluster of issues that arise when a policy question "involves the issue of whether broad categories of persons are to be better or worse off." (Lowi, 1964, 689) The debate over Medicare was in fact cast in the terms of class conflict, of socialized medicine vs. the voluntary "American way," of private enterprise and local control against "the octopus of the federal government." Moreover, though the program most immediately affected the aged, physicians, and hospitals, broad strata of the population were directly or indirectly involved—the families of the aged, all present social security contributors, and the entire health industry.

Not only the themes of the conflict, but the antagonists and their adversary methods illustrate that might be called "class conflict" politics. The dispute over Medicare re-enacted the polarization that characterized earlier fights over national health insurance. The leading adversaries—national business, health, and labor organizations—participated in open communication (though not to their mutual enlightenment) and brought into the opposing camps a

* This formulation of the Lowi scheme owes much to an unpublished paper by Paul Peterson of the University of Chicago: "The Politics of Welfare," 1969.

large number of groups whose interests were not directly affected by the Medicare outcome. In the process, ideological charges and counter-charges dominated public discussion, and each side seemed to regard compromise as unacceptable. In the end, the electoral changes of 1964 reallocated power in such a way that the opponents were overruled. Compromise was involved in the detailed features of the Medicare program, but the enactment itself did not constitute a compromise outcome for the adversaries. In all these respects, Medicare politics differed from the discrete and localized pursuit of pork barrel benefits or the shifting coalitions and compromises of regulatory politics.

Battles like Medicare are fought in public but settled in private. The national pressure groups concerned made enormous and costly efforts to define the dispute over Medicare in ways acceptable to their members. But within the government bureaucracy, there were continuing efforts to articulate and balance these rival claims in the legislation proposed to the Congress. The consultation was sometimes explicit and detailed, as when the AFL-CIO and the Blue Cross Association met regularly with HEW officials during the early 1960s. In other cases, consideration of group interest was tacit and intermittent, particularly in the case of the AMA. Overall, the executive proposals sent to Congress reflected a typical pattern; major compromises were built into Medicare bills proposed by the executive branch, anticipating the pressure group claims that would otherwise have to be balanced in the Congress.

The role of Congress in dealing with policy problems like Medicare is to "ratify the agreement" that arises out of "the bureaucracy and the class agents represented there" (Lowi, 1964, 711). Had Medicare passed in 1964, this characterization of executive preeminence would have been fully warranted; the bill of that year was a hesitantly redistributive version of hospital insurance for the aged, designed to assist the aged but shaped to serve and meet the economic demands of insurance companies and the hospitals as well. The fact that Congress unexpectedly added physician insurance to the program enacted in 1965 represents a departure from the modal processes of redistributive politics, a departure that can be explained by the extraordinary electoral context of 1965. The significant changes in the Administration bill were made almost exclusively in committee deliberations. Minor adjustments arose from Senate debate, none from the House, where the vote on Medicare took place without amendment. The Executive branch was throughout the locus of legislative planning and drafting; the peculiarities of the 1965 Congress should not obscure the patterns of the preceding decade.

The polarization elicited by issues like Medicare shapes the behavior of all the interested pressure groups. Medicare was one of those issues that separates the "money-providing" and "service-demanding" groups in a society—a division which "cuts closer than any other along class lines" (Lowi, 1964, 707, 711). This promotes cohesion among groups that otherwise have much to disagree about; the existence of a common fear promotes a public united front. So, for instance, the conflicting interests of the American Hospital Association (certain to be assisted by Medicare's underwriting of the hospital expenses of the aged) and the American Medical Association (violently opposed to Medicare, despite its members' short-run economic interests) were muted through most of the fight over Medicare. Hospital Association officials felt constrained to take the "health industry's" position against Medicare, though in private (and in meetings with HEW), their willingness to go along with the legislation was apparent. The health industry's public opposition was fused with that of almost every national commercial, industrial, and right-wing group in American politics. The united front of "service-demanders" was equally apparent in the Medicare fight. The ultimate consumers—the aged and their organizations—were sometimes overshadowed in the procession of "liberal" professional, labor, and service organizations championing their cause.

Finally, the processes of Medicare politics involved stabilizing and centralizing conflict in ways characteristic of redistributive disputes (Lowi, 1964, 715). The initiation of Medicare demands in the early 1950s—when the issue was simply whether the social security system would provide 60 days of hospital insurance for its beneficiaries—revealed the pattern of conflict which would follow. Specters of the future—fearful or hopeful—dominated the ideological charges of the national pressure groups. The liberal-conservative split that emerged remained stable throughout, with few defectors as the proposals shifted. The Department of Health, Education and Welfare centralized much of the battle. Congress, whose fiscal committees are short of staff and unequipped to conduct independent research on health affairs, "listened" to the repetitive debates and, in the end, ratified the Administration's bill, adding its own special imprint.

Most Medicare bills did not propose massive redistribution of income, and in this sense the association of Medicare with Lowi's redistributive politics may appear problematic. But the central feature of the Medicare dispute was whether the federal government should engage in whatever limited redistribution Medicare proposals entailed. The fight centered on whether the redistribution was warranted (were the aged needy enough?), the instrument of change (charity or insurance?), and the sources of financing (general revenues or social security taxes?). This redistributive frame of reference determined the shape of the conflict, not the scale of redistribution that would in fact be involved.

Medicare thus appears to be an instance of a much larger class of conflicts in American politics associated with issues of income redistribution and zero-sum political conflicts. Our findings about Medicare can be used, however, to illustrate more than classificatory generalizations. More general questions—involving the structure of power in the United States—are relevant. What was the role of public opinion in this major public policy choice? How influential were pressure groups and whom did they seek to pressure?

The Medicare case illustrates the comparative irrelevance of mass public opinion in federal policy-making (Key, 1961; Bauer *et al.*, 1963). Public support for health insurance under social security declined slightly as remedial proposals were more specifically defined. Polls revealed less support as the probabilities of legislative action increased, a finding comparable to Meranto's (1967) in the case of federal aid to education and consistent with more general conclusions about the nature of mass opinion. When pollsters shift from asking general questions about the need for social action to specific questions about particular remedies, support seems to fragment. In any event, the architects of Medicare never sought public views on legislative details, but rather were after (in V. O. Key's memorable term) a "permissive consensus" (1961). They sought and discovered overwhelming majorities of respondents ready to acknowledge the comparatively severe health and financial problems of the aged. They found substantial majorities willing to support a "solution" to these difficulties through the social security system. In short, they found their "problem" to be credible and their remedial instrument "legitimate." But as one would expect, the polls revealed substantial ignorance of the details of the standard Medicare proposals, and an important and mistaken tendency to assume that Medicare referred to comprehensive medical and hospital insurance (see chap. 4).

The discrepancy between public understanding and the actual Medicare proposal highlights the limited role of mass opinion in this policy area. Public support for "doing something" about the health problems of the aged declined as the question became more specific, from nearly 70 percent support for federal action in general to about 55 percent support for specific Kennedy and Johnson bills. But support, at either level of specificity, did not substantially vary with the prospects of congressional action. No change in public attitude accompanied the enactment of the Kerr-Mills program in 1960. Likewise in 1965 there was no noticeable change in public attitude once electoral changes insured some sort of Medicare legislation.

It might be argued that massive public sympathy with the problems of the aged and mass approval of the social security system were the necessary but not sufficient conditions for the enactment of Medicare. Specifying the impact of such opinion on the policy-making process is, nonetheless, extremely difficult. Those who assume government leaders are limited by what they think the public will buy are perhaps confusing an effort to avoid conflict with groups like the AMA with an attempt to "get around" alleged public preferences. (See the exclusion of surgical benefits from the Medicare proposals from 1958 on, chap. 3.) In the end, public opinion of Medicare's benefits played an indirect and unanticipated role in the expansion of the program. Misunderstandings about the meaning of Medicare—the impression that both physician's and hospital bills would be covered—provided advocates of broader benefits with unexpected political resources. But the way in which this informational discrepancy was taken into account was haphazard, a process of social choice in which critics of Medicare's misleading publicity were used for purposes quite unlike those they accepted.

The long, expensive, and extensive efforts of pressure groups to affect the Medicare outcome should not lead us to confuse the volume or intensity of their publicity with influence. The failure to distinguish group participation from group influence has in fact been a conceptual weakness of the pluralist model of pressure group politics. Lowi (1964, 681) points out that the "proof" of a pluralistic American political structure is all too often entailed by the definitional and conceptual assumptions of the analyst:

> Issues are chosen for research because conflict made them public; group influence is found because groups so often share in definition of the issue and have taken positions that are more or less congruent with the outcomes. An indulged group was influential, and a deprived group was uninfluential; but that leaves no room for group irrelevance.

This conclusion is abundantly illustrated in the attribution of influence to the American Medical Association. Medicare defeats during the 1962–64 period were typically viewed as AMA victories, even though AMA actions were not the chief reason for legislative inaction. To be sure, the AMA did enjoy influence in shaping the Medicare debate. The pattern of Medicare proposals over time illustrated the capacity of the AMA to influence the agenda of discussion and to limit the alternatives policymakers would suggest. Perhaps the most vivid illustration of this preemptive power was the deliberate exclusion of physician insurance from Medicare proposals after 1958. However, if the limits of debate were in part a result of AMA influence, legislative decisions were not. The succession of Medicare defeats arose from congressional power distributions whose effects the AMA could enjoy but whose character the AMA could only marginally affect. The effort to build a coalition in the pre-1965 period took into account AMA objections, but the decisive electoral shift of 1965 illuminated the true basis of past Medicare defeats. The congressional structure—inordinately responsive to Southern Democratic inclinations—was substantially changed for the moment, and Medicare legislation quickly followed. Just as one should distinguish the causes of the enactment of a Medicare bill from the reasons for particular provisions, so one should distinguish the capacity to shape discussion from the ability to produce legislative outcomes.

Much of the alleged power of pressure groups, as shown by recent political science literature, is the product of the imagination and imagery of contending groups. The 1961 battle over Medicare vividly illustrates this process. The Democratic administration helped create an image of a powerful AMA to call attention away from its own incapacity to make Congress (and especially the Ways and Means Committee) do its bidding. Much pressure group effort, in any case, is spent in bolstering group supporters, not changing congressional minds. Such efforts, with the possible exception of regulatory politics, typically involves "inter-reaction with people on the same side" of an issue (Bauer *et al.,* 1963, 398). This was unquestionably the case during the long Medicare conflict, where the two leading group antagonists—the AFL-CIO and the AMA —never had the occasion or inclination for prelegislative bargaining. The executive bureaucracy played a broker's role between these "opposing sides," tacitly incorporating compromises into legislative proposals, particularly in the final stages of enactment. HEW officials like Cohen and Ball consulted labor organizations and the health professions in ways public debate did not allow. The opponents investigated on its merits very little of what each other claimed; there was an overwhelming tendency to bifurcate the universe into friends and enemies and to "learn" only from friends. Pressure groups used the imagined (or real) power of their opponents to rally support for their "side." The massive propaganda efforts of both the AMA and AFL-CIO were never judged by their actual effects on crucial political leaders. Rather, each side indicated the need for solidarity and the seriousness of the conflict by publicizing the propaganda expenditures of its adversary.

It must not be assumed that redistributive social welfare issues alone generate the kind of polarized ideological conflict we have been describing. Redistributive issues may well make up the bulk of such conflicts, but they do not comprise the class. There is a strikingly close parallel between the political processes evidenced in Medicare and those, for example, in public power conflicts in America. Wildavsky (1962) has characterized the latter conflict in much the same way as in the Lowi typology and illustrated by Medicare. The obvious difference between disputes over public power (the public role in electricity, gas, etc.) and federal health insurance should not obscure either the similiar style of conflict or their common ideological roots. Both issues involve the legitimacy of federal action and, by implication, limits on private initiative. In this respect, they differ from pork barrel disputes over how much one area or group or another receives in public expenditures and services. They differ as well from regulatory issues in which, once legislation is effective, the conflicts focus on the burdens and benefits of particular governmental rules. The most bitter fight over Medicare and such public power issues as Dixon-Yates is at the level of principle, not particular burdens and benefits. The question whether the government should be acting at all is central, and in turn calls forth the ideological polarization and national pressure group activity previously discussed. Consider Wildavsky's generalizations about

Dixon-Yates (1962, 304–5) alongside the political processes that characterized Medicare:

1. A very large percentage of the active participants in the controversy divided into well-defined camps with opposing views (the AMA-led opposition versus the AFL-CIO-led proponents). Active individuals who were impartial or uncommitted or who dissented from the two major views were rare.
2. Professional bureaucracies developed with full-time staffs who made a career out of fighting on the issue and there were public figures who made their reputations in this field (e.g., Wilbur Cohen, with long-term social security experts like Ball and Wolkstein, joined by Nelson Cruikshank of the AFL-CIO and William Hutton of the Senior Citizen Organization on one side; and on the other, Dr. Edward Annis of the AMA, and many others, supported by the substantial staffs of the NAM, Chamber of Commerce, American Farm Bureau Federation, etc.).
3. Since the opposing groups had long since been formed, their active members were acutely aware of who was on their side and who was on the opposing team (e.g., the immediate HEW impulse to reject the Byrnes plan in early 1965, chap. 4).
4. Personal contacts were largely restricted to individuals on the same side (the case throughout in Medicare, except for some of the HEW leaders).
5. Having good reason to believe that they had "heard it all before," the disputants were disinclined to listen to arguments on the other side (e.g., participants talking past one another in public hearings throughout the period 1958–65).
7. Opponents had in reserve prepared responses ready to be activated whenever the occasion demanded (e.g., the responses of Medicare proponents to the notion of need, and the familiar arguments against the alleged vices of the social security system).

8. Views on this issue were frequently held with considerable passion, leading to a strong tendency to oversimplify, to regard events and personalities in terms of black and white. One's opponents were regarded as inherently suspect of all kinds of devious actions, while one's supporters were considered to be above suspicion (e.g., the familiar characterization of Cohen as a "Czar" by his critics, and the HEW suspicions of AMA initiatives in 1965).

9. Involvement in the controversey was sufficiently intense for the participants to use a large part of their resources to secure a favorable outcome (e.g., lobbying expenditures, and the proportion of time spent in 1965 on Medicare matters by the top ten HEW officials).

10. While the participants may have had a direct economic stake in the controversy, they came in time to feel that more was involved than money and property. The conflict then took on an ideological hue, with victory or defeat seen in terms of overriding general principles that must not be sacrificed (e.g., the broad appeals on both sides of Medicare to norms of federalism, the "American way," tax policy, the dignity of the aged, the "welfare state," collectivism, etc.).

The issues which generate such broad ideological polarization range beyond health insurance and public ownership of power plants. Studies of the legislative dispute over federal aid to education have recently documented similar features (Munger & Fenno, 1962; Meranto, 1967; Eidenberg & Morey, 1969). Past disputes over public housing have activated similar antagonists and methods of antagonizing (Friedman, 1968). But not all, or even most, political conflicts assume this form; generally it is when the legislative issue is the broad redistribution of power and income (money, services, and authority), that the quest for initiative or for veto coalititons generates the processes of polarization. The site and agents of such conflict clearly vary from issue to issue. Sometimes the dispute is lodged in the executive (Dixon-Yates) and extensively covered

by the media. In other cases, conflict and concessions are brought
out in congressional committees, with the executive branch playing
a somewhat more passive role (public housing and some welfare
legislation). Within Congress, issues vary as to whether amendment
and substantial adjustments take place through floor action (education legislation and appropriations, for example) or in committee.
The important point is not the site of such conflicts, but the parties
that fight them out and the issues that generate them. What constitutes the limits of this class of policial conflicts is an important empirical question that individual case studies cannot answer. One
may not assume from the evidence given here that redistributive issues are always class-based and ideological, or that idiological polarization always arises about the likely redistributive impact of a
given policy. But one can conclude that explicitly redistributive issues strikingly generate the sort of conflict that characterized Medicare politics.

Neither Wildavsky nor Lowi, however, tell us anything about the
typical outcome of such conflicts. The analysis of the content of ideologically divisive policies does not logically follow from generalizations about processes of conflict. An independent inquiry is required concerning the kinds of policy outcomes one might expect
from the disputes Wildavsky and Lowi have described.

Medicare and the Character of American Social Policy

This section will briefly compare Medicare's programmatic structure with other American public policies, particularly other social
welfare programs. This concern with the content of public policy
responds to an impulse that other American political scientists have
noted and encouraged. Ranney (1968, 3) rightly contends that "at
least since 1945 most American political scientists have focused
their professional attention mainly on the *processes* by which public
policies are made and have shown relatively little concern with their
contents." Ranney is at pains to distinguish programmatic intentions and practices from the consequences they produce, to separate

a policy and its outcome. The relation between policies (their intended objects, goals, programmatic practices) and political outcomes (affected persons, principles served, and subsequent practices) is an empirical issue of great interest. The study in this book has taken Medicare policy (in the above sense) as its subject and cannot hope to comment extensively on the consequences that followed its adoption and implementation. Nonetheless, my present purpose is to consider the policy contents of Medicare not for what they tell us about American political processes but to compare the nature of that policy itself with others.

There is no need to repeat my previous descriptions of the Medicare program: its noncomprehensive health insurance benefits, regressive financing, aged beneficiaries, centralized and nondiscretionary administration, and nonmeans-tested eligibility features. Rather, two central issues warrant comment here. The first is the appropriateness of the classificatory criteria that permitted such a description; the second is the generality of this type of programmatic result.

Policies may be described by their beneficiaries (the poor, farmers, widows, etc.), their financing (regressive, proportional, progressive), their administrative structure (centralized or decentralized, discretionary or nondiscretionary), their source of entitlement (earned or unearned), the extent of their departure from past practices (radical or incremental). Little is gained from debate over which descriptive set is most useful; that depends upon the purpose of the inquirer. But much is gained—for those interested in the burdens and benefits of American public policy—by characterizing who is to benefit from and who is to administer a given policy. These questions can be applied to any policy at any level of government. They thus permit generalizations about programs that are quite different in the goods or services they distribute.

Friedman (1969) has used such a scheme in characterizing American housing policy in the recent past. He identifies two social welfare policy types as "middle-class" and "charity" programs. Such emotive terms are not necessary to observe that Medicare rep-

resents the former type and that the Medicare debate centered on
the choice between these two models:

Criteria	Middle-class program	Charity program
Beneficiaries	Broad demographic unit, not selected by test of means	"Needy" persons selected by test of means
Benefits	Earned, noncomprehensive for given problem	Given, not earned, and more comprehensive
Financing	Regressive, as with earmarked Social Security taxes	General revenues, more progressive source
Administration	Centralized, nondiscretionary and clerk-like, with highly developed rules of entitlement	Discretionary, decentralized

Not all social policies represent one or the other of these polar
types, but some, such as the social insurance provisions of the Social Security Act of 1935 and Medicare, are pure middle-class programs. In such programs, "benefits tend to be a matter of right; eli-
gibilities are earned; benefits are restitutionary; the means-test is
avoided" (Friedman, 1969, 247). The characteristics of "charity
laws" like Medicaid or Kerr-Mills "are flatly reversed." A review of
the contrast between the Forand and Kerr-Mills proposals would
support the interpretation that these two conceptions of appropriate
social policy were at stake.

The extent to which other social policies fall into this dichoto-
mous pattern can only be answered through investigation. Exceptions come immediately to mind. The old-age assistance program in
California, for instance, is widely known for the dignified way in
which beneficiaries are selected and for the clerk-like character of
program administration. The income-tested veterans pension is,
likewise, a means-tested program that has little of the degrading
and discretionary character commonly associated with public assist-

ance, and is an example of centralized federal programs for "needy" persons. But the issue is not whether exceptions exist, but what constitutes the general patterns of social policy. This case study attests only to the plausibility of the Friedman classification.

Friedman is interested as well in the determinants of each type of social welfare legislation. Public assistance—particularly general relief at the local level and federal-state assistance to families with dependent children (AFDC)—typify what have been termed "charity" programs. That is not meant to suggest that such programs are charitably run, but that means-tested programs are associated with local discretion and general tax funds. Friedman suggests that the effort to elicit wide support for programs that avoid the connotations of "welfare" almost inevitably, in American politics, produce middle-class legislative models. The designated clientele (needy persons rather than a demographic unit) is the causal key. Programs for both the rich and the poor make means tests less relevant, and local administration less crucial. Restitutionary programs are legitimated by past acts, not present income; they avoid the moral choices between deserving and undeserving recipients by designating recipients in terms of past contributions or neutral demographic attributes. Finally, the clientele theory assumes that the particular type of benefit (cash or kind) does not determine the form of the policy, or its likely character over time. There are, Friedman would argue, two major types of "social welfare policy," not distinctive health, housing, education, and cash-transfer policies.

The foregoing remarks apply primarily to types of social welfare laws, not patterns of policy consequences. Not only may implementation deviate from statutory intention, but statutes and programs may distribute different types of benefits. Edelman (1964) has rightly distinguished between the symbolic burdens and benefits which statutes may provide and the tangible assistance (and deprivation) which operating programs in fact distribute. Not all statutes are strictly enforced, and "preambles to legislation" can be used to "symbolize concern and hoodwink people with symbolic reassurance that all will be well once the law is on the books" (Mitchell, 1969, 162). The passage of Medicare unquestionably involved such symbolic reassurance. But its implementation distributed intended financial benefits to the aged even though all might not be well once the law was on the books. In addition, however, there were substantial unintended beneficiaries from the programmatic practices of the Social Security Administration and the health insurance industry.

The most striking development was the extent to which Medicare benefited those who opposed it most. Medicare was advocated as an insurance measure, not as an instrument of reform in the organization and delivery of personal health services. Though physician services were typically excluded from Medicare proposals, the AMA was Medicare's most hostile critic and the most serious symbolic loser from its enactment. But physicians have received substantial income supplements from the Medicare program thus far, as have critics in the nursing home and hospital industries. The cooperation of health businesses was required, and Medicare was clearly intended to assist hospitals (through the improved capacity of their aged patients to pay) and insurance companies (relieved of the financially onerous task of insuring the aged at low premiums). But the scale of such assistance (and its extension to physicians) was unappreciated by most of those who participated in the legislative process. Those who think health groups wrung such concessions as a price of legislative cooperation confuse intended with unintended consequences, and explicit with tacit bargaining. Most of the generous features of Medicare were attempts to forestall difficulties, not respond to them. And the price of such generosity, four years later, prompted the Department of Health, Education and Welfare to warn about the "extreme urgency of the [health cost] situation, [and] to encourage steps to arrest the inflation that is paralyzing us." Such price inflation was not intended, even by those in the Johnson Administration who most understood that the bitter Medicare bill must be sweetened for its opponents in the health industry.

Since the enactment of Medicare, the prices of hospital and physician services have risen markedly. The arrangements for paying physicians were more generous than their lobbyists might have expected even had they participated in negotiations on methods of payment (Marmor, 1968). Physician fees have risen between 5 and 8 percent per year since the start of the program; physician incomes, nearly 11 percent per year (Somers, 1968). These increases have made American physicians among Medicare's most prominent beneficiaries. This result was not only unintended by Medicare proponents, but largely unanticipated in the course of the legislative struggle over the 1965 bill. This development suggests caution in describing public policies primarily by the benefits and beneficiaries specified in law.

The implementation of Medicare illustrates another important distinction between legislative action and policy content. When issues are moral and symbolic, as in legislative struggles over the redistribution of important resources, a great variety of attentive publics are aroused. In Medicare there were active national pressure groups representing large numbers of Americans directly or indirectly involved in the health and financial circumstances of the aged. When questions arose about Medicare's administration, some attentive groups become financially interested parties, the producer groups, involved in the production and delivery of health services. The aged remained active, of course. and along with the representatives of the AFL-CIO, have sat on advisory bodies set up by the Social Security Administration at congressional behest. The hospital, nursing home, laboratory, and physician representatives nonetheless predominate. This administrative confrontation is a relatively new experience for Medicare's Social Security Administration. SSA has "never had to deal," said one official rather sadly, "with hostile pressure groups at the administrative level." The nature of conflict changes when the political question turns to who receives tangible benefits. The Social Security system—distributing cash directly, for the most part—has never had to rely on the cooperation of hostile industries in anything but tax collection. It is in administrative politics that well-organized producers are at an advantage; their interest in symbolic issues carries over to practical struggles in ways one does not predict of general reform groups and consumer organizations. The Social Security Administration was thus unprepared to deal with economic pressure groups, especially those which, though ideologically opposed to social insurance, were nonetheless desperately interested in the benefits actually distributed by a program whose initiation they in other contexts strongly opposed.

Bibliographical Citations

Books

ANDERSON, ODIN (1968), *The Uneasy Equilibrium,* New Haven: College & University Press.

ANDERSON, RONALD and ODIN ANDERSON (1967), *A Decade of Health Services,* Chicago: University of Chicago Press, 122ff.

BAUER, RAYMOND, A. ITHIEL DE SOLA POOL, and LEWIS DEXTER (1963), *American Business and Public Policy,* New York: Atherton Press.

BURROW, JAMES G., (1963), *AMA: Voice of American Medicine,* Baltimore: Johns Hopkins Press, pp. 244–47, 288–89.

CANTRIL, HADLEY (1952), *Public Opinion: 1935–1946,* Princeton: Princeton University Press, pp. 439–44.

CORNWELL, ELMER E. Jr. (1965), *Presidential Leadership of Public Opinion,* Bloomington: Indiana University Press, 240–41.

DAVIS, MICHAEL M. (1941), *America Organizes Medicine,* New York: Harper & Brothers, 167–68.

EDELMAN, MURRAY (1964), *The Symbolic Uses of Politics,* Urbana: Illinois University Press.

125

EIDENBERG, EUGENE and ROY D. MOREY (1969), *An Act of Congress,* New York: W. W. Norton & Company, Inc.

FEINGOLD, EUGENE (1966). *Medicare: Policy and Politics,* San Francisco: Chandler Publishing Co.

FRIEDMAN, LAWRENCE (1968), *Government and Slum Housing,* Chicago: Rand McNally and Company.

FROMAN, LEWIS A. Jr. (1968), "The Categorization of Policy Contents", in Austin Ranney, Ed., *Political Science and Public Policy,* Chicago: Markham Publishing Company, chap. 3.

GREENFIELD, MARGARET (1966), *Health Insurance for the Aged: The 1965 Program for Medicare,* Berkeley: Institute of Governmental Studies, University of California, 88, 26–28.

HAMILTON, RICHARD F., (forthcoming), *Class and Politics in the United States,* chap. 2.

HARRIS, RICHARD (1966), *A Sacred Trust,* New York: New American Library.

KELLEY, STANLEY Jr. (1966), *Professional Public Relations and Political Power,* Baltimore: Johns Hopkins Press, 60, 70–71, 77.

KEY, V. O. (1961), *Public Opinion and American Democracy,* New York: Knopf.

LASSWELL, HAROLD (1958), *Who Gets What, When, How,* Cleveland: The World Publishing Company.

MERANTO, PHILIP (1967), *The Politics of Federal Aid to Education in 1965,* Syracuse: Syracuse University Press.

MITCHELL, JOYCE M. and WILLIAM C. (1969), *Political Analysis and Public Policy,* Chicago: Rand McNally & Co., 162.

MUNGER, FRANK J. and RICHARD F. FENNO (1962), *National Politics and Federal Aid to Education,* Syracuse: Syracuse University Press.

MUNTS, RAYMOND (1967), *Bargaining for Health: Labor Unions, Health Insurance and Medical Care,* Madison: University of Wisconsin Press.

PETERS, CLARENCE A., Ed., (1964), *Free Medical Care,* New York: H. W. Wilson Co., 38.

RANNEY, AUSTIN, Ed., (1968), *Political Science and Public Policy,* Chicago: Markham Publishing Company.

ROSE, ARNOLD M. (1967), *The Power Structure,* New York: Oxford University Press, 422.

SALISBURY, ROBERT H. (1968), "The Analysis of Public Policy: A Search for Theories and Roles" in Austin Ranney, ed., *Political Science and Public Policy,* Chicago: Markham Publishing Company, chap. 7.

SOMERS, HERMAN and ANNE SOMERS (1961), *Doctors, Patients, and Health Insurance,* Garden City: Anchor Books.

SOMERS, HERMAN and ANNE SOMERS (1967), *Medicare and the Hospitals: Issues and Prospects,* Washington, D.C.: The Brookings Institution, 136.

WILDAVSKY, AARON (1962), *Dixon-Yates: A Study in Power Politics,* New Haven: Yale University Press, 5–6, 304–5.

Articles

ALLISON, GRAHAM T. (1968), "Conceptual Models and the Cuban Missile Crisis," paper presented at the 1968 Annual Meeting of the American Political Science Association, Washington, D.C., Sept. 2–7, 1968, 1. *(The American Political Science Review,* September, 1969).

ANDERSON, ODIN W. (1951), "Compulsory Medical Care Insurance, 1910–1950," *The Annals of the American Academy of Political and Social Science,* 273 (Jan. 1951): 106–13. Reprinted in Eugene Feingold (ed.), *Medicare: Policy and Politics* (San Francisco: Chandler Publishing Co., 1966).

BALL, ROBERT M. (1964), "The American Social Security Program," *New England Journal of Medicine,* 270 (Jan. 30, 1964): 232–36.

COHEN, WILBUR J. (1960), "Health Insurance Under Social Security," reprinted from the *American Journal of Nursing,* 60 (April, 1960): 5.

COHEN, WILBUR J. and ROBERT M. BALL (1965), "Social Security Amendments of 1965: Summary and Legislative History," *Social Security Bulletin* (Sept., 1965), 5.

FRIEDMAN, LAWRENCE (1969), "Social Welfare Legislation," *Stanford Law Review*, 21, (Jan., 1969): 247.

GALLUP, GEORGE (1965). "Majority Backs Medical Care of Aged Through Social Security," *Public Opinion News Service* (Jan. 3, 1965).

HYDE, WOLFF, *et al.* (1954), "AMA: Power, Purpose, and Politics in Organized Medicine," *Yale Law Journal* (May, 1954).

LOWI, THEODORE (1964), "American Business, Public Policy, and Political Theory," *World Politics*, 16 (1964).

MARMOR, THEODORE (1968), "Why Medicare Helped Raise Doctors' Fees," *Transaction* (Sept., 1968), 4.

MAYER, MARTIN (1949), "The Dogged Retreat of the Doctors," *Harper's* (December, 1949), 36.

MANLEY, JOHN F. (1965), "The House Committee on Ways and Means: Conflict Management in a Congressional Committee," *American Political Science Review*, 59 (Dec., 1965): 927–39.

Nation's Business. (Sept., 1962); cited in American Medical Association, *Federalized Health Care for the Aged* (1963), 52–53.

New Republic. (1962), "Evaluation of Ways and Means Democrats, First Session, Key Votes—87th Congress" (October 27, 1962).

New Republic. (1965), "New Deal II," 152 (March 20, 1965).

Newsweek (May 8, 1961), 103.

New York Herald Tribune, June 9, 1961, 11.

New York Times
    (1, 1961) *New York Times,* Feb. 10, 1961.
    (2, 1961) *New York Times,* Feb. 19, 1961.
    (3, 1961) *New York Times,* Feb. 11, 1961.
    (4, 1961) *New York Times,* April, 1961.
    (5, 1961) *New York Times,* Jan. 5, 1961.
    (6, 1961) *New York Times,* April 5, 1961.

(1965) "Medicare's Progress," *New York Times,* March 25, 1965.

RICE, DOROTHY P. and LOUCELLE A. HOROWITZ (1968), "Medical Care Price Changes in Medicare's First Two Years," *Social Security Bulletin* (Nov., 1968).

SCHECTER, MAL (1968), "Emergency Medicare and Desegregation: A Special Report," *Hospital Practice,* (July, 1968), 14–19, 63–64.

Wall Street Journal, Feb. 8, 1965.

American Medical Association Publications

(1961) *A National Legislative Program for County Medical Societies: Operation Hometown* (Chicago: American Medical Association, 1961).

(1, 1963) *The Case Against the King-Anderson Bill (H.R. 3920),* Statement of the American Medical Association before the Committee on Ways and Means, House of Representatives, 88th Congress (Chicago: American Medical Association, 1963), 17.

(2, 1963) *Federalized Health Care for the Aged* (Chicago: American Medical Association, 1963), 52–53.

(1965) "Why Eldercare Offers Better Care than Medicare," American Medical Association (March, 1965).

Congressional Hearings

(1, 1961) *Health Services for the Aged Under the Social Security Insurance System (H.R. 4222), Hearings Before the Committee on Ways and Means,* House of Representatives, 87th Congress, 1st Session, July–Aug., 1961.

(2, 1961) Testimony of Secretary Ribicoff, *Health Services for the Aged Under the Social Security Insurance System, Hearings Before the Committee on Ways and Means,* House of Representatives, 87th Congress, 1st Session, I (July–Aug., 1961).

(1965) *Trends in Quantity and Quality of Health Insurance Coverage Among the Aged, Executive Hearings, Ways and Means Committee,* House of Representatives, 89th Congress, 1st Session (1965), 40–44.

Congressional Reports

(1963) *The Kerr-Mills Program, 1960–1963; Report of Subcommittee on Health of the Elderly,* Special Committee on Aging, U.S. Senate, 88th Congress, 1st Session (Oct., 1963), 1–4.

(1, 1965) *Social Security Amendments of 1965; Report of the Committee on Ways and Means of H.R. 6675,* 89th Congress, 1st Session, Report No. 213 (Washington, D.C.: U.S. Government Printing Office, 1965), 61–62.

(2, 1965) *Ibid.,* 54.

(3, 1965) *Summary of Major Provisions of House of Representatives 6675, The Social Security Amendments of 1965 as Agreed to by the House, Senate Conference Committee,* Committee on Ways and Means, 89th Congress, 1st Session (July 21, 1965), 4.

Legislative Reference Service, Education and Public Welfare Division. (1963) *The Federal Government: Role in Providing Medicare to the Citizens of the U.S.,* Library of Congress (Washington, D.C.: U.S. Government Printing Office, 1963).

Congressional Quarterly Service Publications

(1, 1965) *Congress and the Nation: 1945–1964* (Washington, D.C.: Congressional Quarterly Service, 1965), 1113, 1116.

(2, 1965) *Ibid.,* 4, 7.

(3, 1965) *Legislators and the Lobbyists* (Washington, D.C.: Congressional Quarterly Service, (1965), 77–78.

(4, 1965) *Congressional Quarterly,* Weekly Report, June 25, 1965.

(5, 1965) *Congressional Quarterly,* Weekly Report, XXIII (Jan. 1, 1965).

HEW Publications

(1959) *Health Manpower Source Book,* Public Health Service Publication no. 263, sec. 9 (Washington, D.C.: U.S. Government Printing Office, 1959), 26–29.

(1962) *The Health Care of the Aged,* Social Security Administration (Washington, D.C.: U.S. Government Printing Office, 1962), 22–32.

(1964) *Chart Book of Basic Health Economic Data,* Public Health Service Publication no. 3 (Washington, D.C.: U.S. Government Printing Office, 1964), 22.

(1, 1965) *Background Book on Hospital Insurance for the Aged Through Social Security—H.R. 1,* Unpublished Data, HEW, 1965, IX-B-6.

(2, 1965) HEW Memorandum, Alanson W. Willcox, General Counsel to Wilbur J. Cohen, Assistant Secretary (May 21, 1965), Re: H.R. 6675—Douglas Amendment on Hospital Specialists.

(1, 1967) *A Report to the President on Medical Care Prices* (Washington, D.C.: U.S. Government Printing Office, 1967), 19, 31.

(2, 1967) "Current Data from the Medicare Program," Health Insurance Statistics, HEW (Nov. 20, 1967).

(3, 1967) *A Report to the President on Medical Care Prices* (Washington, D.C.: U.S. Government Printing Office, 1967), 2

(1968) *The Drug Users* (Washington, D.C.: U.S. Government Printing Office, 1968).

(1969) *A Report on the State of the Nation's Health Care System,* (July 10, 1969).

Other Unpublished Sources

ASKEY, VINCENT, M. D. (1961), "Aging, Medicine, and Kerr-Mills," Address delivered before the California Medical Association, Los Angeles, California (May 1, 1961).

BRAY, HOWARD—Staff Member (1965), "Memorandum on Important Defects in H.R. 6675 Currently Under Discussion in the Senate Finance Committee," (May 20, 1965).

COHEN, WILBUR J.—Assistant Secretary HEW (1965), "Memorandum for the President," March 2, 1965.

MILLS, WILBUR D. (1964), "Financing Health Care for the Aged," Address before Downtown Little Rock Lions Club, Little Rock, Arkansas (Dec. 7, 1964), Duplicated in *HEW Background for the 1965 Legislative Session,* IX B-1, Jan. 25, 1965.

QUEALY, WILLIAM H. Minority Counsel (1965), "Memorandum to Ways and Means Republicans," Jan. 17, 1965.

SOMERS, ANNE (1968), "Total Financing of Health Care: Past, Present, and Future."

VINYARD, DALE (1972), "The Senate Committee on the Aging and the Development of a Policy System," paper delivered at the Political Science Section of Michigan Academy, East Lansing, Michigan (March, 1972).

WOLKSTEIN, IRWIN (1968), Letter to T. R. Marmor, Dec. 11, 1968.

Sources, Acknowledgments, and Further Readings

This study rests upon a variety of sources: interviews, congressional hearings and debates, the personal files of government officials and pressure group spokesmen, newspapers, magazines, and published books and articles on medical care, welfare legislation, and American politics.

For the evolution of the Medicare issue, four books were most useful: Stanley Kelley's *Professional Public Relations and Political Power* (Baltimore: The Johns Hopkins Press, 1956); Herman and Anne Somers' broad account of the medical care industry up to 1960, *Doctors, Patients, and Health Insurance* (Washington, D.C.: The Brookings Institution, 1961); Richard Harris' history of Medicare politics, *A Sacred Trust* (New York: The New American Library, 1966); and Eugene Feingold's *Medicare: Policy and Politics* (San Francisco: Chandler Publishing Company, 1966).

Detailed studies of the character of American physicians and their professional organizations can be found in: Elton Rayack's *Professional Power and American Medicine: The Economics of the American Medical Association* (Cleveland: The World Publishing Company, 1967); James G. Burrow's *AMA: Voice of American Medicine* (Baltimore: The Johns Hopkins Press, 1963); Corrine

133

Gilb's *Hidden Hierarchies: The Professions and Government,* (New York: Harper & Row, 1966); Oliver Garceau's *Political Life of the AMA* (Cambridge: Harvard University Press, 1941); and Hyde, Wolff, *et al.* "AMA: Power, Purpose and Politics in Organized Medicine," *Yale Law Journal* (May, 1954).

For the history of the growth of voluntary health insurance and the controversy over government health insurance see: James Howards Means' *Doctors, People, and Government* (Boston: Little, Brown and Company, 1953); James Rorty's *American Medicine Mobilizes* (New York: W. W. Norton and Company, 1939); Somers and Somers' *Doctors, Patients, and Health Insurance;* Odin Anderson's *The Uneasy Equilibrium* (New Haven: College Publishing Company, 1968); and Franz Goldman's *Voluntary Medical Care Plans in the United States* (New York: Columbia University Press, 1947). The early administrative experience of the Medicare program is presented in Herman and Anne Somers' *Medicare and the Hospitals* (Washington, D.C.: The Brookings Institution, 1967).

The special problems and circumstances of the aged are extensively reported in the following books: Peter O. Steiner and Robert Dorfman, *The Economic Status of the Aged* (Berkeley: University of California Press, 1957); Ethel Shanas, *Family Relationships of Older People: Living Arrangements, Health Status and Family Ties of Those Aged 65 and Over, As Reported by the Aged, the Persons to Whom They Would Turn in a Health Crisis, and the General Public* (Chicago: Health Information Foundation, 1961); and *Financing Health Care of the Aged: A Study of the Dimensions of the Problem* (Chicago: Blue Cross Association and American Hospital Association, 1962). Several special governmental reports dealing with the problems of aged are available, including: The U. S. Senate Committee on Labor and Public Welfare, *The Aged and the Aging in the United States: Summary of Expert Views,* 86th Congress, 1st Session, June 1959; The Senate Committee on Labor and Public Welfare, Subcommittee on Problems of the Aged and Aging, *Action for the Aged and Aging: A Report,* Senate Report No. 128, 87th Congress, 1st Session, March 28, 1961; The Senate Subcommittee on Aging, *Background Facts on the Financing of the Health Care of the Aged: Excerpts from the Report of the Division of Program Research, Social Security Administration, Department of Health, Education, and Welfare,* 87th Congress, 2nd Session, 1962; HEW-SSA, Division of Program Research, *The Financial Position of the Aged,* by Lenore A. Epstein, Research and Statistics Note No. 1, 1962; Senate Subcommittee on Aging, *Developments in Aging, 1959 to 1963,* Senate Report No. 8, 88th Congress, 1st Session, 1963; HEW-SSA, *Income Security Standards in Old Age,* by Lenore A. Epstein, Research Report No. 3, 1963; and HEW-SSA, Division of Research and Statistics, *Estimated Expenditures for Medical Care of Persons Aged 65 and Over,* Research and Statistics Note No. 3, 1963.

For the congressional responses to Medicare and executive and pressure group activities, a wide range of sources was employed. *The Congressional Quarterly* and the published Medicare hearing before the Ways and Means Committee (1958–65) give basic descriptions of the treatment of bills within the Congress. The American Medical Association's weekly *AMA News* provides a useful index to doctors' responses to Medicare proposals. *The New York Times* and *The Wall Street Journal* were the main newspaper sources.

Interviews provided much valuable information, and I should like here to express my appreciation for the courtesy extended me. (All of the words of those interviewed are not directly quoted for obvious reasons of properiety.) Interviews with HEW personnel in 1966 included: Wilbur J. Cohen, Undersecretary of HEW; Robert Ball, Commissioner of Social Security; Irwin Wolkstein, SSA Staff; Dean Costen. Deputy Undersecretary of HEW: Ralph Huitt, Assistant Secretay of HEW; Dr William Stewart, Surgeon General of the Public Health Service; William Fullerton, then of the Administration on Aging; Morris Older, SSA Staff Physician Reimbursement under Medicare; and Thomas Tierney, Head of the SSA Bureau of Health Insurance. Among the interviews conducted with congressmen and staff the most extensive included: Representatives Wilbur Mills and Al Ullman; William Quealy, Minority Counsel, House of Representatives Committee on Ways and Means; and Jay Constantine, Staff, Senate Committee on Finance. Interest group leaders interviewed included: Dr Ernest B. Howard, now Executive Vice-President of the American Medical Association; Leo Brown, the AMA's Director of Communications; Walter McNearny, chief executive of the Blue Cross Association, and his staff associate Steven Sieverts; and Tom Mura of the Blue Shield Association. Particularly informative were interviews with reporters who covered Medicare developments, especially Arlen Large of *The Wall Street Journal* and John D. Morris of *The New York Times*. Access to the personal files of Wilbur J. Cohen provided an extensive collection of materials on the origins of Medicare.

Discussion and correspondence with Professor Odin Anderson, Dr Osler Peterson, Sidney Lee, and Dr Lester Breslow were very helpful. Valuable criticism of various portions of the manuscript was provided by Martha Derthick, R. Harrison Wagner, Peter Townsend, Adrian Sinfield, Herman Somers, Robert Eyestone, Raymond Munts, Ira Sharkansky, Murray Edelman, and A. D. Tillet. Ken Dolbeare, Richard Hamilton, Lawrence Friedman, Graham Allison and Theodore Lowi, were particularly helpful in the final revisions of chapter 6.

For students interested in pursuing this topic further, a useful guide to the differing legislative proposals since 1952 can be found in Margaret Greenfield's *Health Insurance for the Aged* (Berkeley: Institute of Governmental Affairs, 1966). The National Center of Health Statistics, The Public Health Service, and the *Social Security Bulletin* have published medical and financial profiles of the aged that are valuable and easily available.

Those interested in congressional responses to controversial social legislation in the 1960s should compare this case with the fate of federal aid to education bills: Frank J. Munger and Richard F. Fenno, *National Politics and Federal Aid to Education* (Syracuse: Syracuse University Press, 1962); Philip Meranto's *The Politics of*

Federal Aid to Education in 1965 (Syracuse: Syracuse University Press, 1967); H. Douglas Price, "Race, Religion, and the Rules Committee: The Kennedy Aid to Education Bills," in Alan F. Westin (ed), *The Uses of Power* (New York: Harcourt, Brace and World, 1962). Instructive comparisons from the areas of public welfare and national housing legislation include: Gilbert Y. Steiner, *Social Insecurity: The Politics of Welfare* (Chicago: Rand McNally, 1966); and Lawrence Friedman, *Government and Slum Housing* (Chicago: Rand McNally, 1968). Harry Eckstein's *The English Health Service* (Cambridge, Mass.: Harvard University Press, 1948) can be read as a parallel analysis of social policy-making abroad, and provides comparative illustration of those distinctively American features of medical politics revealed by the Medicare conflict.

A basic survey of the literature on the structure and character of the United States Congress can be found in William J. Keefe and Morris S. Ogul, *The American Legislative Process: Congress and the States* (Englewood Cliffs, N. Y.: Prentice-Hall, 1964). Further readings on the Congress are also provided by Robert L. Peabody and Nelson W. Polsby, *New Perspectives on the House of Representatives* (Chicago: Rand McNally, 1963). In the June, 1968 issue of the *American Political Science Review,* L. Froman gives a contemporary characterization of the dominant features of the Congress. For a description of the conventions of the House of Representatives, see Clem Miller's *Member of the House* (New York: Scribner's, 1963). A discussion of congressional-executive relations can be found in Nelson W. Polsby's *Congress and the Presidency* (Englewood Cliffs, N. J.: Prentice-Hall, 1964). For an authoritative study of the Ways and Means Committee, consult John F. Manley's "The House Committee on Ways and Means: Conflict Management in a Congressional Committee," *The American Political Science Review,* 59 (Dec., 1965): 927–39, and his longer work, *The Politics of Finance: The House Committee on Ways and Means* (Boston: Little, Brown and Company, 1970).

Glossary

139

AFL-CIO   A national federation of craft and industrial unions.

American Association for Labor Legislation   A group of lawyers, academics, and other professionals, active during the years 1915–20, who tried to get model medicare bills through several state legislatures.

Blue Cross Association   Non-profit hospital insurance organizations loosely affiliated with the American Hospital Association and its state members.

Blue Shield Plans   Non-profit medical insurance organizations, sponsored by state medical societies, whose boards of directors are composed mostly of physicians.

Closed-rule   A procedure of the House of Representatives under which no amendments are permitted and debate is limited, on a bill for which a vote is to be taken.

Co-insurance   The proportion of health charges for which patients are responsible.

Conference committee   An ad-hoc committee created to adjust differences between House and Senate versions of a bill.

Deductibles   The payments that patients must make before their insurance company is responsible for charges.

Discharging a bill   A congressional rule which enables a majority of the members of the House to compel a committee to release its hold on a bill or resolution and to send it to the floor. A discharge petition must be submitted and an appropriate time schedule followed.

Federal Security Agency   The Agency created in 1939 to oversee the Social Security Board, the Public Health Service, and the Office of Education. In 1953 it was replaced by the cabinet-rank Department of Health, Education and Welfare.

Floor-manager The congressman who guides the bill through floor action in either the House or Senate.

Floor stage The period after a bill is discharged from committee and put on the legislative agenda. Bills reach the floor stage when they are considered by the entire body of either the House or Senate.

Grant-in-aid Money given by the national government to the states if the latter are willing to meet conditions specified by Congress. The national agencies that administer the funds require the states to submit their plans for advance approval.

Intermediaries The middle-men who handle transfers of money. In the case of Medicare, the insurance companies, Blue Cross and Blue Shield Plans have been designated as fiscal intermediaries.

Mark-up The formal review and revision of a bill in committee before it is released for floor action.

Medical vendor payments Money paid to dispensers of medical goods and services.

Party whip The party leader whose major duties are to keep party members informed of legislative proceedings and to muster support when a vote is being called.

Premium payments The financial payments (monthly, yearly) which purchase a contract of insurance.

Programmatic majority A majority in Congress favoring a particular bill, as opposed to a party majority.

Public Health Service The federal agency charged with planning and coordinating health services and facilities and located within the Department of Health, Education, and Welfare.

Recommit a bill The procedure whereby a bill before either the House or Senate is sometimes sent back to the committee in which it originated for further consideration and alteration. An indirect way to delay or defeat legislative proposals.

Reported out of committee   The legislative stage following passage of a bill by a committee when it is placed on the legislative agenda of either the House or Senate.

Rider   An amendment tacked onto a bill which is well on its way to passage but which is really a separate piece of legislation. A device to circumvent opposition.

Roll-call vote   A formal vote in which the preferences of individual Congressmen are officially recorded.

Speaker of the House   The presiding officer of the House of Representatives and the acknowledged leader of the majority party.

Sponsor   The legislator who introduces a bill in either house of the Congress.

Index

143